THE NHS IN SCOTLAND

The NHS in Scotland

The legacy of the past and the prospect of the future

Edited by
CHRIS NOTTINGHAM
Centre for Contemporary History
Glasgow Caledonian University

Ashgate

Aldershot • Burlington USA • Singapore • Sydney

Published by
Ashgate Publishing Limited
Gower House
Croft Road
Aldershot
Hampshire GU11 3HR
England

Ashgate Publishing Company
131 Main Street
Burlington
Vermont 05401
USA

Ashgate website: http://www.ashgate.com

British Library Cataloguing in Publication Data
The NHS in Scotland : the legacy of the past and the
    prospect of the future
    1.National Health Service in Scotland - History 2. Medical
    care - Scotland - History
    I.Nottingham, Chris
    362.1'09411

Library of Congress Control Number: 00-132841

ISBN 0 7546 1276 7

Printed in Great Britain by
Antony Rowe Ltd, Chippenham, Wiltshire

Contents

List of Contributors

Maarten van Bottenburg was co-founder and managing partner of Research Bureau Diopter until 1998. He now is managing partner/director of Diopter - Janssens & Van Bottenburg. Among several books and many articles, he wrote: *Verborgen competitie. Over de uiteenlopende populariteit van sporten* [Hidden competition; On the differential popularities of sports] (Amsterdam 1994), *Aan den arbeid! In de wandelgangen van de Stichting van de Arbeid* [To work! Behind the scenes of the Labour Foundation] (Amsterdam, 1995) and *Zorg tussen staat en markt. De maatschappelijke betekenis van de Ziekenfondsraad 1949-1999* [Care between state and market. The social impact of the Sickness Fund Council 1949-1999] (Zutphen 1999, with Geert de Vries and Annet Mooij).

John Curnow is Director of Public Health and Chief Administrative Medical Officer, Orkney Health Board. He is also Senior Clinical Lecturer in Public Health Medicine at the University of Aberdeen and Senior Vice President of the Royal Environmental Health Institute of Scotland. His professional interests include infectious diseases, in particular gut pathogens and E.coli O157, medical aid for humanitarian crises, disaster medicine and military medicine. He is heavily involved in the development of remote and rural medicine particularly with new models of care being undertaken in Orkney.

Marguerite Dupree is a Senior Lecturer and a core staff member of the Wellcome Unit for the History of Medicine at the University of Glasgow. She holds a Wellcome Trust University Award during which she plans to undertake the project outlined in this paper. She is the editor of *Lancashire and Whitehall: the Diary of Sir Raymond Streat 1931-1958* and is the author of *Family Structure in the Staffordshire Potteries 1840-1880*. She is also the author of a number of articles in the social history of medicine particularly on the relationship of families and hospitals in nineteenth century British cities, on the use of computers in the history of medicine and on aspects of the development of the medical profession in Britain in the nineteenth and twentieth centuries. In addition to her work with Anne

Crowther for their forthcoming book, *Lister's Men: Medical Lives in the Age of Surgical Revolution*, she is currently working on a book, *Hydropathy, Medicine and Society in Scotland 1840-1950* with James Bradley and Alastair Durie.

Rona Ferguson is a Research Assistant in Glasgow Caledonian University and is studying for a doctorate in the departments of Social Science and Nursing & Community Health. Her thesis is a history of district nursing in Scotland based largely on oral testimony. She has published on the history of women in medicine and on district nursing in Scotland most recently 'Nurse Jenny a'Thing. Recollections of life on the district' in Johanna Bornat, Robert Perks & Paul Thompson (eds.) *Oral History of Health and Welfare* (Routledge, 1999).

Jacqueline Jenkinson is a Lecturer in History at the University of Stirling. Her current research, which was funded by the ESRC is on Scottish health policy 1918-1948. Her publications include a book on Scottish Medical Societies, and she co-authored the history of Glasgow Royal Infirmary. She has recently published a contribution on Scottish health policy and practice, 1918-1948, to the collection *Improving the Public Health*, 1998.

Ronald Johnston is a Research Fellow in Scottish History at the University Strathclyde. He has published extensively on the history of occupational health and safety and is currently writing a book with Arthur McIvor, *Dust to Dust: the Asbestos Tragedy in Scotland* (Tuckwell Press, 2001). He is the author of *Clydeside Capital* (Tuckwell Press 2000).

Susan McGann is the Archivist of the Royal College of Nursing based in Edinburgh. She is the author of *The Battle of the Nurses: eight leaders in the development of professional nursing, 1880-1930*, Scutari Press 1992, many articles on the history of the RCN and 'Archival sources for research into the history of nursing', *Nurse Researcher*, 5 (2), 1997/98.

Arthur McIvor is a Senior Lecturer in History at the University of Strathclyde. He has published extensively on the history of occupational health and safety and is currently writing a book with Ronnie Johnston, *Dust to Dust: the Asbestos Tragedy in Scotland* (Tuckwell Press, 2000). His previous publications include *Organised Capital* (Cambridge University

Press, 1996), and *A History of Work in Britain 1880-1950* (Macmillan, 2000).

Hugh McLachlan is Reader in Sociology in the School of Social Sciences at Glasgow Caledonian University. He has published extensively in a range of areas in the philosophy of the social sciences. He is currently heavily involved in writing on issues of medical ethics, most notably on commercial surrogacy. He is a regular contributor to the *Journal Of Medical Ethics*.

Annet Mooij was co-founder and managing partner of Research Bureau Diopter until 1998. She is now owner and director of the Research Bureau Mooij Onderzoek. She has published numerous books and articles, such as *Out of Otherness. Characters and narrators in the Dutch venereal disease debates, 1850-1990* (London 1998), *Zorg tussen staat en markt. De maatschappelijke betekenis van de Ziekenfondsraad 1949-1999* [Care between state and market. The social impact of the Sickness Fund Council 1949-1999] (Zutphen 1999, with Geert de Vries and Maarten van Bottenburg) and *De polsslag van de stad. 350 jaar academische geneeskunde in Amsterdam* [The city's pulse. 350 Years of academic medicine in Amsterdam] (Amsterdam, 1999).

Chris Nottingham is Senior Lecturer in Politics at Glasgow Caledonian University, and Visiting Research Fellow of the Contemporary History centre in the University of Amsterdam. He publishes mainly in the history of health and welfare politics. His book, *The Pursuit of Serenity. Havelock Ellis and the New Politics* was published by Amsterdam University Press in 1999.

Fiona O'Neill is Lecturer in the Department of Nursing at the University of Leeds. She has just completed a Ph.D. thesis in the Department of Politics of the University of Birmingham on the involvement of nurses in the policy process. Before turning to politics she trained and practised as both a general and psychiatric nurse. She has published articles in the Journal of Nursing Management, Parliamentary Affairs and Contemporary Political Studies. Her most recent work is 'Ideas Across an Ocean, The Internal Market reform of the NHS' in David Donowitz (**ed.**) *Policy Transfer and*

Public Policy Making, Learning from the American experience, Open University Press (April 1999).

David Player After a distinguished and unusually varied medical career David became Director of the Health Education Board of Scotland and later Director General of the Health Education Council. He is a former chair of the Public Health Alliance and has published articles in the Health Bulletin, the Journal of Health Education and the Scottish Trade Union Review.

Alistair Tough is currently Resident Consultant on Records Management to the Public Sector Reform Programme of the Government of Tanzania. He was previously the Archivist of the Greater Glasgow Health Board. He has been a Fulbright Fellow at Stanford University, Snell Visitor at Balliol College and a Bentley Fellow at Michigan University. In the British General Elections of 1992 and 1997 he contested the Clydebank and Milngavie and Stirling constituencies respectively as a Liberal Democrat. He is the author of *African medical history. A guide to personal papers in Rhodes House Library, Oxford* (Bodleian Library, 1998) and co-author of *Selecting clinical records for long term preservation* (Glasgow Wellcome Unit, 1993).

Geert de Vries works in Diopter Bureau of Social Research (Amsterdam) and Amsterdam School of Social Research (University of Amsterdam). He has (with his co-author Maarten van Bottenburg) just completed a study of the 'Ziekenfondsraad' (Dutch Sickness Fund Council), *'Zorg tussen staat en markt: de maatschappelijke betekenis van de Ziekenfondsraad, 1949-1999'* [Health Care between State and Market: The Social Impact of the Sickness Fund Council, 1949-1999] (January 1999). He is co-editor of the Amsterdams Sociologisch Tijdschrift and the Netherlands Journal of Social Science.

Foreword

The papers in this volume represent a wide range of perspectives and encompass diverse points of view. They are however united in the core problem which they address. They were originally conceived as contributions to a conference in Glasgow Caledonian University organised by the Centre for Contemporary History on the first fifty years of the NHS in Scotland. In the course of our discussions on that day three themes emerged. Firstly there was a sense of impatience that many of the reflections which the fiftieth anniversary of the Service had inspired had been so uncritically celebratory. While most would agree that the NHS had represented a considerable advance on what preceded it, this should not preclude clear analysis of the Service's deficiencies as they had emerged over time, nor restrict discussion of possible future improvements. The NHS can never be regarded as an end in itself. In reality the Service has been in a state of perpetual change throughout its existence and this will continue to be the case. If the NHS is to deliver the highest quality of service possible to the greatest number, this will require a constant adaptation to developing technologies, standards and needs

The second theme was that of public health. All discussions of the NHS lead at some point to the consideration of how far, in its emphasis on cure, the Service has tended to neglect the work of prevention. Any adequate health policy should surely address the social and behavioural factors which tend to make people ill in the first place. Even if the NHS had proved admirable in many of its aspects, it is not difficult to identify deficiencies in this. Our contributions reflect the long battle for the public health perspective, a developing tragedy caused by its neglect, and some thoughts on how beneficial change might come about in the future.

In Scotland, the celebration of the fifty years of the NHS was in some sense overshadowed by the certainty of imminent change. The third theme was therefore suggested by the impending transfer of democratic responsibility for the Service from Westminster to a devolved parliament in Edinburgh. While none of those involved in that process are committed to a revision of the fundamentals of NHS, there is widespread recognition this must inevitably result in change of some sort. The history of the health services in Scotland is somewhat neglected and is certainly worth developing for its own sake, but it would be unrealistic at this juncture to ignore its pertinence to this major theme of public debate. The question of whether there is anything particular in the past and current provision of health services in Scotland, some characteristic set of attitudes, on which the Scottish parliament and executive can begin to forge a distinctive approach is of fundamental political importance, not only for the future of the NHS but for the whole devolution settlement. Arguments about the NHS have always aroused deep political emotions, never more so than in the past two decades, and it is safe to predict that they will continue at the same level of intensity. While no work could hope to anticipate the whole of that coming debate, we hope that these papers do begin to define some of the issues and suggest some of the opportunities.

In editing a book of this nature one runs up a good many debts of gratitude. First I must thank the contributors not only for their splendid papers but also for delivering them in good time and in a respectable form. I can safely leave the papers to speak for themselves, but I must mention two authors whose contributions demanded special efforts. Firstly Geert de Vries, who having just completed a major study of the equivalent fifty year period in the development of health care in the Netherlands, has outlined for us his thoughts on parallels with the NHS. He has moreover, produced his paper in attractive English. Anyone who is surprised to find an article about the Dutch experience appearing in a volume specifically concerned with Scottish issues will quickly see in Geert's paper the pertinence of the experience of other systems to our current debates. Secondly I wish to express special thanks to John Curnow. One weakness of the original conference was a failure to sufficiently reflect the immense diversity of the NHS in Scotland, surely one of its most characteristic features. While we dealt with the particular problems of the major urban areas, the difficulties of delivering health care in the remote regions to match the promise of the NHS of equal standards, were not adequately addressed. I am therefore very grateful to John for finding time in his busy life to share his ideas with us.

I must also thank all those who helped with the original conference, in particular Willie Thompson and Catriona MacDonald of the Centre for Contemporary History, and Kevin Dalton and Yvonne Brown for so cheerfully sacrificing their time. Anyone who undertakes an enterprise of this kind will understand how important institutional support is to success and in this respect I feel a special debt of gratitude to Elaine McFarland, as

Head of the Division of History and Politics, to David Walsh, as Head of the School of Social Sciences, and to Gordon Dickson, as Dean of the Faculty of Health, for support, advice and assistance. Happily all of them have since moved upwards.

Finally I must record a debt of gratitude to my wife Annet, not only for all the usual forbearances which academics with a project demand of their nearest, but also for considerable help in the editing of the volume. Only she and I will ever fully appreciate the literal truth of the statement that it would not have been possible without her.

1. Scottish Health Policy 1918-1948 - Paving the Way to a National Health Service?

JACQUELINE JENKINSON

Introduction - Creation of the Scottish Board of Health

The Scottish Board of Health (SBH) was established in 1919 and became the umbrella unit for all the existing components of Scottish health administration, including the Local Government Board for Scotland, the Scottish Insurance Commissioners, and the Highlands and Islands (Medical Services) Board (established in 1894, 1911 and 1913 respectively). The Highlands and Islands Medical Service (HIMS) which now came under SBH control was a distinctive and uniquely Scottish entity: a public medical service established in 1913 to provide medical care for those in the remote regions of Scotland who had often lacked the basic medical services of general practitioner, consultants and clinic facilities due to the difficult nature of their environment. The main aim of the HIMS was to provide a subsidised medical service to the largely crofting communities of the remote Highlands and Islands, an area covering almost half of Scotland, with a population less than one-fourteenth of the country. Many of the special services contemplated in the initial legislation of 1913 were not immediately introduced due to wartime circumstances and it was under the SBH that the HIMS flourished. For example, as the scheme developed in the 1920s, general practitioner and nursing services were improved and staffed surgical centres established.

The creation of a Scottish Board of Health in 1919 was not a simple matter. Dr. Christopher Addison the first Minister of Health, piloted the Ministry of Health Bill through Parliament in the months immediately following the end of World War One. Addison rejected the idea of including Scotland in the Health Bill on the grounds that the formation of separate Ministries of Health for Scotland and Ireland would complicate the Bill's passage and involved potential constitutional dangers by raising the issue of federalism. Addison made clear his views in a letter to the Scottish Secretary, Robert Munro in March 1918: '... a strong section of Scottish opinion will be directed towards making this Bill the occasion for effecting a constitutional change in the Government of Scotland...'[1]

However, Addison's worst fear was that wrangling over Scottish and Irish health and local government reforms would delay, or defeat, the proposals for a new health ministry. Consequently, he restricted his plan for a Ministry of Health to England and Wales. Addison formally disassociated himself from the proposal by Scottish Secretary Robert Munro to the War Cabinet that the existing Scottish Local Government Board and the Scottish Insurance Commission be united in a single health office and that a new Parliamentary Under Secretary to the Scottish Office be appointed. Yet, the Scottish Secretary's plan won the day in Cabinet discussion. One reason why the Cabinet gave in to Munro's pressure and ignored Addison's recommendations was the representations from outside agencies in support of a Scottish clause to the Health Bill:

> In Scotland, the volume of opinion in favour of the Bill was very strong, and important deputations from local authorities and labour organisations were unanimous in pressing upon the Secretary for Scotland the urgency of the matter.[2]

Viewed in this light, Scotland could be considered as fortunate in gaining its own health administration. Yet the creation of a separate health administration did not necessarily signify a devolved Scottish health policy. In fact, among the ranks of Scottish MP's there were fears that external control by the Scottish Office, based at Dover House in London, would affect adversely the new Health Board's abilities to solve the pressing problems of Scottish health. Joseph Johnstone Coalition Liberal MP for East Renfrewshire, went as far to state that Scottish people distrusted 'the influence of the Scottish Office in London, and they want to work this Department apart from the paralysing influence of the Scottish Office...'[3] This suggests that there were perceived difficulties in the new system in allocating responsibility between central and Scottish government, as well as a possible divide between the Whitehall-based Scottish Office and the Edinburgh-based Scottish Board of Health.

Consultation and Policy Formulation

Under the new Scottish Board of Health (SBH), four Consultative Councils were created as a vehicle to canvass interested opinion from around Scotland on the shape and functions of the new State health agency. One of these was the Consultative Council on Medical and Allied Services which represented the interests of the medical profession. The Council's Interim report (the MacAlister Report) entitled 'a Scheme of Medical Service for Scotland' was issued in November 1920. In essence, the Report recommended that the health service of the nation should be based on the family as the normal unit of health care and that the family doctor (general practitioner) be the focus of this health care. The MacAlister Report recommended the provision of a complete medical service under the SBH through the extension of national health insurance to all dependants of those currently insured. The existing services were to be expanded to cover all forms of health care required, including preventive monitoring of the whole community. The MacAlister Report proposed that the new co-ordinated medical service should function under the control of a unified system of local authorities.[4]

The Report of the Consultative Council on Medical and Allied Services was received at the end of 1920 for earnest consideration by the SBH.[5] However, the Report's submission was rapidly followed by a directive from the Treasury restricting planned expenditure in many areas of government for the financial year 1921-1922 and the recommendations of the MacAlister Report were not implemented. Government financial restriction may not have been the sole reason for inaction on the Report. For example, the Report itself was not universally well received by the medical profession. The MacAlister Report of 1920 was an innovative, wide ranging document, which influenced later thinking on the extension of public medical services.[6]

Despite the inability of the SBH to act on the MacAlister Report, the Scottish Consultative Councils continued to meet and produce new policy proposals. In 1921, the Consultative Council on Local Health Administration and General Health Questions issued an interim report advising the reduction in the number of public health authorities in Scotland by creating larger units.[7] In 1923, the Council produced a final report on the reform of local government health administration. Its main suggestion was to amalgamate small inefficient local authorities into larger units based on county councils and burghs of over 50,000 population.[8] The recommendations of the Report were not immediately put into operation, but were broadly incorporated into the clauses of the Local Government (Scotland) Act of 1929.[9]

The Local Government Act of 1929 was the culmination of a series of proposals to reorganise the Scottish system of local government to allow Scottish local authorities to administer public health more effectively. Under the new legislation, Parish Councils were abolished, small burghs lost their autonomous powers and county councils were set up. The reform was very much on the lines of the SBH Consultative Council's earlier proposals. The recommendations of the MacAlister report of 1920 for an enhanced public medical service were based on the assumption that local authorities would be reformed and rationalised. The 1923 Health Administration Consultative Council's suggestions to reduce the number and greatly increase the size of local authorities, were now put into operation.

Administrative Overhaul

The organisation of the Scottish Board of Health was itself the subject of persistent review in the 1920s. The SBH was not run by an administrative civil service like the Ministry of Health, but by a group of expert individuals and career administrators, who, (according to Scottish Secretary John Gilmour in 1928) often brought forward inappropriate and unrealistic policies. This led Gilmour during the 1928 reorganisation of offices debates in Parliament to express in plain terms the problems which (he felt) had arisen in the SBH policy formulation since its creation in 1919:

> We have heard much about the technical experts. I am not averse from, nor will any regulation, which I make prevent intercourse between the experts and those responsible for administration... . Parliament must direct policy and control the experts. We know that the expert is often carried beyond the bounds of what is possible in finance or in relation to actual affairs. Is the expert always to have his way? ... if the medical man had his way, he might possibly impose upon Parliament and the country a system - eminently desirable no doubt in itself - but so extravagant, or so much in advance of the times, that Parliament could not tolerate it.[10]

Gilmour's argument is clear. Medical and other expertise within the Board system could lead to the favouring of policy with a strong bias towards extended public medical services. Although not specifically mentioned, the 1920 MacAlister Report could fit easily into Gilmour's scathing attack on SBH policy initiatives. This independent strain of opinion within the Board system ran contrary to the existing central government administrative system which had developed under a professional civil service The difference in administrative structure meant that from its very inception there were calls to overhaul the Scottish Board system along Whitehall civil service lines and various attempts throughout the 1920s to reorganise the SBH. Before the summer recess in 1923, a Reorganisation of Offices (Scotland) Bill was brought before Parliament by the then Scottish Secretary, Viscount Novar.[11] Although the Bill failed, as did later Reorganisation Bills of 1924 and 1927, the long-awaited reorganisation of the Board system in Scotland finally occurred in 1928. One reason for the delay in implementing structural reform was the high level of domestic political support for the existing Scottish Boards, including the Board of Health.

For example, when the third Reorganisation Bill was put forward in 1927 it was not widely supported in Parliament. William Adamson Labour MP for West Fife[12] feared that the Government was attempting to subordinate Scottish administration to Whitehall to a far greater extent than previously had been the case and to ... remove from Scotland practically the last vestige of independent government and nationhood, and to have its centre in London.[13] The Reorganisation Bill of 1927 did not go beyond a Second Reading and a further Reorganisation Bill was introduced by new Scottish Secretary Gilmour in February 1928. In order to deflect the criticism levied at the previous Bill that control was to be shifted to Whitehall, Gilmour inserted a clause specifying that the new Departments were to be situated in Edinburgh.

In Parliament, the Labour opposition expressed the fear that even if Whitehall was not to be the physical location of the new Scottish Departments, power would invariably rest in London. Tom Johnston Dundee Labour MP (and a future Scottish Secretary) stated:

> Now we find this Government... deliberately attempting to take away the detailed administration of public affairs in Scotland from bodies of presumably skilled men [sic], who have been nominated because of their knowledge of those particular affairs. It is proposed that the direction of these affairs should be handed over to men who, whatever examinations they might have passed in Oxford or Cambridge, have not proved their

fitness to conduct those great businesses upon which the lives and happiness of our people depend.[14]

The transformation in 1928 of the Health, Agriculture and Prison Boards into Departments more directly under the control of the Secretary of State aroused misgivings that control of Scottish government affairs within Scotland was at risk. There was also the question of a political divide, as Conservative governments attempted to reorganise the Scottish Boards and were steadily resisted by Labour (and sometimes Liberal) opposition. However, local autonomy was not completely removed, as the 1928 reorganisation allowed the new Departments a degree of independence from the Secretary of State. The absence of shared appointments and any interchange of staff between the Departments also fostered an independent outlook and local loyalty. The powers of the Office of the Scottish Secretary to effect further administrative changes were also constrained by the need to seek Parliamentary approval through the established legislative process.

Although the SBH was itself replaced by a Department of Health for Scotland in 1929, little changed as regards the system of external policy advisers. The work of the Consultative Councils in Scotland continued. For example, in 1933, the Scottish Consultative Council on Medical and Allied Services produced a Report on Hospital Services[15] which recommended a co-ordinated hospital service. However, as with the MacAlister Report of 1920 this recommendation was set aside until the time was more auspicious for wide ranging health reforms.

The Cathcart Report, 1936

Further far-reaching proposals were recommended by another advisory committee set up by the DHS. In 1933, the Scottish Health Services Committee was established. It reported three years later. The 1936 Cathcart Report,[16] built on the recommendations of the 1920 Consultative Council on Medical and Allied Services (MacAlister Report). Indeed, the Cathcart Report explicitly referred to the earlier report as influencing its enquiry. The Cathcart Report proposed a National Health Service for Scotland with a new comprehensive and co-ordinated structure of medical and allied services, and an extension of the general practitioner services to the whole population. It planned for the co-ordination of general practitioner services with existing medical services, such as maternity and infant welfare and school health.

Reaction to the Report was mixed. The Cathcart Report gained equivocal support from the medical profession. For example, the Scottish BMA supported the notion of increased responsibility for the general practitioner, as did the Royal Colleges.[17] However, within the medical profession there was also strong resistance to the idea of a state medical service involving government payments for general practitioners. The possibility of a comprehensive state-funded health service was raised in the evidence given before the Cathcart Committee, with both the Scottish Trade Union Council and Glasgow Corporation supporting the idea of a full-time salaried medical service. This proposal was not included in the main report itself, but was raised in a minority recommendation.

In Parliament, the Conservative-dominated National Government did not welcome the Cathcart Report findings with enthusiasm. Scottish Secretary Godfrey Collins glossed over it in the discussions on the annual estimates of the DHS in July 1936. Lack of Government support combined with the predominance of the policy of economy, ensured that of the Cathcart Report recommendations, only the suggested scheme of an extended maternity service was put into operation. Yet the ambitious Cathcart Report helped lay the groundwork for the operation of a distinctive health service suited to Scotland's specific health needs post-1948.

The 1937 Maternity Services (Scotland) Act owed much to the findings both of the 1936 Cathcart Report and the 1935 Report of the DHS Committee on Maternal Morbidity and Mortality. The persistence of high maternal mortality rates in Scotland throughout the 1930s (see Table 1 and Figure 1) made this one area where government action was regarded as essential, despite the need to economise in public expenditure. The intention of the Act was to create a public maternity service under local authority control, which would allow midwives, general practitioners and consultant obstetricians to combine to provide comprehensive maternity care. Under the new legislation, payment for the new service was to be recovered by local authorities only where women were in a position to afford such payments. Inability to pay was no longer to be a barrier to an extended range of maternity care.

The DHS investigations of 1935 and the Cathcart Report revealed that existing Scottish maternity services were woefully inadequate. The differences between maternal care in Scotland, and England and Wales and the detrimental effect this had on Scottish maternal mortality was raised in Cabinet by Scottish Secretary Sir Godfrey Collins in May 1936. Collins stressed that maternal mortality remained significantly higher in Scotland than in England and Wales. He stated that under the existing maternity services midwives only attended 25 per cent of childbirth cases (in comparison with 60 per cent in England); and that in consequence, doctors continued to play a disproportionate role in maternity cases (with few positive results). Collins also noted that geographic factors had to be given particular consideration in framing new maternity legislation, in view of Scotland's mix of dense urban conurbations and scattered rural communities:

> The practical impossibility of applying arrangements - e.g., ante-natal and postnatal clinics - suited to an industrial or urban area, to districts such as the Highlands and Islands, and the varying conditions in regard to maternity practice even as between different urban areas make it essential to frame proposals sufficiently broad and elastic to ensure the development by local authorities of services suited to the circumstances of their areas.[18]

The Maternity Services (Scotland) Act of 1937 was only partially operated in the shorter-term due to the reluctance among doctors to become involved in a scheme, which involved taking direction and (insufficient) payment from local authorities. Only a limited implementation of the scheme could be claimed by the outbreak of the Second World War. However, by June 1943 schemes were in operation in forty-one of the fifty-five Scottish local authorities.

Other elements in the Cathcart Report influenced wartime proposals for a new National Health Service. For example, a sub-committee of the Cathcart Committee considered health services in the Highlands and Islands. While the sub-committee reported that hospital services in the region remained inadequate, (despite initiatives such as the development of the Northern Infirmary, Inverness) and that much had still to be done regarding nursing services in the area,[19] overall, the sub-committee was well satisfied with what had been achieved in the region. In fact, the sub-committee proposed that the HIMS, with its unique blend of local and central government control, should be used as a model for the wider application of extended public medical services elsewhere in Scotland. The proposals were incorporated in the main Cathcart Report and re-appeared in the National Health Service White Paper of 1944.[20] These proposals were dropped after the war, when the idea of a comprehensive health service run by the local authority was rejected in favour of a centrally administered medical service.

Despite the existence of the HIMS and a succession of radical proposals emanating from DHS-sponsored committees, Scotland continued to have one of the worst health records of the industrialised world in the inter-war years. Much time and effort had gone into making detailed proposals to improve and extend the health services to meet the needs of the people in a variety of reports including both the MacAlister and Cathcart Reports. Yet few suggestions were put into operation by the end of the 1930s: the overriding desire for economy in public services was partly behind this inaction. However, the great changes in the government of the nation's health, which occurred, between 1946-1948 were conducted in the wake of the Second World War - the most expensive undertaking the country had ever witnessed. This suggests that it was political will (or lack of it), which determined the level and nature of public health provision in the country at any given period.[21]

Wartime Innovations in Social Medicine

A positive wartime development with regard to Scottish health care was the creation of an extended, and in some respects preventive, State-sponsored hospital service. Such a service had been suggested for a number of years, specifically in the Report on Hospital Services by the DHS Consultative Committee on Medical and Allied Services in 1933. In the event of war breaking out it was assumed there would be huge numbers of civilian wounded. In the spring of 1938, the DHS surveyed the hospitals in Scotland and other buildings, including hotels and public schools, to see where beds could be obtained for the expected air raid casualties. In response to such enquiries, the Emergency Medical Service (EMS) scheme was established in autumn 1938. Through the related Emergency Hospital Scheme, the EMS greatly increased hospital accommodation, expanded the provision of specialist facilities and services, and brought together the various types of hospital authority on a regional basis. The Civil Defence Act of 1939 (Section 50) laid responsibility on the DHS to prepare hospital facilities for civilian casualties as a result of enemy action. Later responsibility was accepted by the Scottish Secretary for the treatment of service personnel in the event of their numbers being too great for the service hospitals to cope. The expected number of casualties never arrived, and by 1941 schemes were put into operation by Wartime Scottish

Secretary, Tom Johnston, to make use of the increased hospital and nursing home capacity which had been created.

In some respects, wartime Scottish Secretary Tom Johnston (acting under advice from the DHS) can be viewed as a pioneer of the coming National Health Service. In 1941, Johnston introduced the voluntary hospitals waiting list scheme (building on suggestions first discussed by his predecessor John Colville in late 1939). This innovative wartime measure made possible the transfer of patients from voluntary hospital waiting lists to emergency war hospitals. Johnston secured the co-operation of both the voluntary hospitals and general practitioners for this unique measure. The scheme allowed patients to be taken from the long voluntary hospital waiting lists for treatment at the new, largely unused wartime casualty hospitals. The charge to the voluntary institutions was 30/- per patient (irrespective of length of stay). At first, the take-up of this scheme was poor, as it was initially restricted to short-stay surgical patients: In 1941, 2,000 cases from voluntary hospital waiting list were treated in EMS hospitals. In January 1942, the scheme was extended to include all but chronic cases. During 1942 the numbers treated rose to 8,000.[22] Speaking in the House of Commons in 1945, Johnston described the positive achievements of the scheme in reducing voluntary hospital waiting lists and of its immediate benefits to thousands of patients.[23] By the middle of 1945, 32,826 patients had been taken off voluntary hospital waiting lists to be treated in the EMS hospitals.[24]

The 1941 voluntary hospital waiting lists initiative was followed by the creation of the Supplementary Medical Service Scheme in January 1942. This scheme used the hospitals of the Clyde Valley area as centres for the recuperation of hard-pressed wartime industrial workers.[25] The Clyde Valley hospitals took patients from the nearby Clyde Basin area, (that is, the City of Glasgow and the counties of Lanark, Renfrew and Dunbarton) which housed 40 per cent of Scotland's insured workforce. Much wartime industrial production was carried out in this area. The DHS view was that the health of industrial workers in this part of Scotland could be safeguarded by drawing upon the full range of public and personal medical services, which had come under central control for the first time due to the wartime emergency. Tom Johnston took advantage of the recently constructed (and fortunately under-used) troop hospitals, which came under his control as part of the Emergency Medical Service Scheme, to extend their facilities for specialist services to civilian war workers.

This Supplementary Medical Service Scheme or Clyde Basin experiment (as it was also known) was an experiment in preventive medical care which involved close co-operation between family doctors, consultants and hospital services. With this initiative, the need for preventive health care, first outlined in the 1920 MacAlister Report, was at last recognised (albeit in a wartime emergency situation). The scheme was initially confined to young industrial workers in West Central Scotland aged fifteen to twenty-five who were in a debilitated state. The focus on younger workers in part reflected an official intention to tackle the growing wartime incidence of tuberculosis.[26] Later, the scheme was extended to cover workers of all ages in all Scottish counties (except the Highlands). Patients were referred by their own doctors for assessment by the Regional Medical Officers and examined by consultants, where necessary; if a further examination was required, they were admitted to an EMS hospital, or sent for convalescence to one of the auxiliary hospitals.

In 1943, the British Medical Journal reviewing the recently-published DHS report on its wartime initiatives in social medicine, Health and Industrial Efficiency, commented approvingly on the Supplementary Medical Service Scheme:

> The Englishman may well have begun to wonder why Scotland has been able to initiate a number of experiments in social medicine since war began, and the Department of Health ... acknowledges that the accommodation available in EMS hospitals has made much of the work possible. The Clyde Basin experiment, for example - remarkable because it is directed to maintaining the health and efficiency of young civilian workers - was made practicable because beds were available at two base hospitals - Law and Killearn - in addition to convalescent-home accommodation.[27]

In July 1942, the DHS supplied details of the Clyde Basin experiment for the information of the War Cabinet's Inter-Departmental Committee on Social and Allied Services (the Beveridge Committee). The Beveridge Committee considered public health issues as an integral part of its remit, and took evidence on Scottish health provision as well as National Health Insurance and Contributory Pensions Scheme and Public Assistance. In the DHS Memorandum the Health of War Workers, on file among the Beveridge Committee papers, the preventive element of the scheme was given great emphasis:

The experiment is designed to safeguard the health of young war workers - largely by preventive measures. It was inaugurated by the Secretary of State issuing to all 'panel' doctors in the area of the Clyde basin a letter in which he appealed for their help in protecting the health of the workers, especially those between the ages of 15 and 25. He suggested that doctors should take the chance whenever possible of overhauling young patients, and intimated that, to help them with those cases, the Department's Regional Medical Service was available.[28]

The publication of the Report on Social Insurance and Allied Services on 1 December 1942 dramatically changed the climate of opinion regarding peacetime health services. The Beveridge Report[29] recommended the creation of a single unified social security scheme and in addition, proposed the creation of a free, comprehensive health service. Assumption B of the Report outlined the health requirements of the new Social Services system: Comprehensive health and rehabilitation services for prevention and cure of disease and restoration of capacity for work, available to all members of the community. This stated recommendation bears more than a passing resemblance to the goals of the Clyde Basin experiment (Supplementary Medical Service Scheme) operated by the DHS.

The future shape of Scottish hospital provision became a topic for wartime discussion as part of the wider debate on post-war reconstruction. In October 1943, the DHS Office Committee made a set of proposals, which underlined their commitment to social medicine:

(a) the Supplementary Medical Service Scheme should continue until the introduction of the Comprehensive Health Service;
(b) that the kind of service now given under the Supplementary Medical Service should become a permanent feature of preventative medical service.[30]

These recommendations were later underlined in June 1945, when new Scottish Secretary Joseph Westwood (in recognition of the importance of the extended hospital facilities which had been introduced during the war), pledged to continue to make the additional wartime beds available for the use of the Scottish population. At the start of the war Scotland had 35,331 hospital beds (21,248 in voluntary and 14,083 in local authority hospitals), by the end of the war the total had risen to 48,101. By this measure, a net addition of 12,970 beds remained in use post-war in Scotland. In mid-1946, the DHS announced that the EMS hospitals would continue to be administered by the Department pending the reconstruction of the health services. In other words, both the DHS and the Scottish Secretary were committed to a State-run hospital service (including its preventive aspects) for Scotland.

Initiated by wartime requirements, the Emergency Medical Service in Scotland was in peacetime incorporated into a comprehensive service under the direction of the DHS and the Scottish Secretary of State. This transformation was a dynamic initiative, but it was not clear that these wartime ventures would become long-term, hence the DHS were careful not to look beyond immediate post-war need in preserving the Emergency Medical Service (hospital and ancillary) provision.

A Distinct Entity? The NHS in Scotland

The change in government as a result of the Labour landslide at the July 1945 election also brought an alteration in direction as far as the planned health service for the nation was concerned. A centrally controlled health service was now envisioned rather than a comprehensive municipal service based on the local authority as the unit of control. The legislative measures introduced by the new Minister of Health, Aneurin Bevan in March 1946 and in December 1946[31] by Scottish Secretary Joseph Westwood were significantly altered from those proposed by the wartime National Government. Both Bills sought to nationalise all hospitals and remove health services such as maternal and infant welfare from the local authorities. The Bills also sought to emphasise the development of health centres, centralise control over the distribution of doctors around the country and introduce payment of general practitioners.

During his introduction to the Second Reading of the NHS (Scotland) Bill in December 1946, Joseph Westwood made great play of the continuities of the new measure with the recommendations of the 1936 Cathcart Report. Westwood had been a member of the Cathcart Committee and he stated that he and six other people (on the eighteen member Cathcart Committee) had at the time signed a reservation stating their belief that a free, comprehensive general practitioner service available to all was the best way forward for the Scottish health services. Despite Westwood's reminiscences, a crucial recommendation contained in the Cathcart Report, that the general practitioner should be the lynchpin to any reorganised health service, was ignored in the new legislation.

Westwood emphasised that Scottish health policy had a long history of State intervention and funding of health care, focused mainly in the Highlands and Islands. He identified the Highlands and Islands Medical Service as a forerunner of the planned NHS: I am often asked what will become of that service in future under proposals contained in this Bill... What, in fact, is happening is that the Bill is extending to all Scotland many features hitherto operating in the Highlands and Islands.[32] Westwood noted that not a single representation against the NHS (Scotland) Bill had been received from doctors working in the HIMS. By implication, those already working in a proto-State medical service saw the benefits of the new proposals for the whole country. The same could also be said for those working under the EMS wartime hospital arrangements in Scotland. The National Health Service (Scotland) Act was passed on 21 May 1947. A little over a year later, on 5 July 1948, the National Health Service came into operation.

Conclusion

In wartime Scotland, the EMS and its Hospital Scheme was an unrivalled success. By contrast, there was no attempt to create a State-run hospital service based on the EMS elsewhere in Britain. As a result, when proposals were put forward for a comprehensive health service which would include all hospitals, there was less resistance to this in Scotland than elsewhere in the United Kingdom and effective integration was achieved in a relatively painless manner. The work of the EMS hospital services had shown both the medical profession and the public that a State-run hospital service could function smoothly.

The Second World War gave fresh impetus to investigations into the state of public medical care. The War also provided the opportunity to experiment with an expanded range of state health services, especially in Scotland. Yet, in the wake of emergency measures, and the debate on a comprehensive health service which they partly fuelled, there was also clear continuity with pre-war DHS policy initiatives and debates, with inter-war reports on health provision, and the existing Highlands and Islands Medical Service having a formative role to play in shaping the new universal system.

The NHS Scotland legislation seemed to be a compromise between the need for a comprehensive health service, which followed to a great extent the 1946 NHS Act for England and Wales, and yet did not neglect the traditions of independent Scottish health policy. The latter was maintained through the creation of Scottish Hospital Management Boards.

These had more devolved powers than their counterparts, the English Hospital Management Committees, and crucially, included the government of the prestigious University teaching hospitals. Also, in Scotland, overall administrative control was placed in the hands of the Scottish Secretary and not the local authorities, as was the case in England.

This chapter has illustrated a number of areas relating to policy making and implementation where the Scottish health administration, while itself undergoing change, was able to follow its own agenda. Indeed, this agenda, as a whole, was influenced by particular areas of concern in the health of the Scottish population. The continued vibrancy of the Scottish Consultative Councils in the 1920s and 30s, the creation of distinct policies on maternal welfare (although not completely successful), and the setting up of the Clyde Basin experiment of preventive hospital care, illustrate the continued distinctiveness of Scottish health administration. After a difficult inception, and some inter-war re-organisation, Scottish health services administration was fully based in Edinburgh by the 1930s. After 1948, the NHS in Scotland maintained its separate identity from the Ministry of Health in London, despite the pressures of administrative centralism.

Notes

1. Public Records Office (PRO), Kew, London PRO MH78/70 Letter from Addison to Munro 19 Mar. 1918.
2. PRO CAB 26/1 Home Affairs Committee, 3rd meeting, 18 July 1918, 'Ministry of Health Bill'.
3. Hansard Parliamentary Debates, House of Commons (HOC), 1 Apr. 1919 vol. 114, column 1146.
4. Scottish Board of Health (SBH) Interim Report of Consultative Council on Medical and Allied Services *A Scheme of Medical Service for Scotland* (1920), pp.6-7.
5. *SBH Second Annual Report, 1920* [Cmd 1319] HMSO, (1921), p.257.
6. Such as in its call for unified local authorities which eventually came with the Local Government (Scotland) Act of 1929.
7. *Glasgow Medical Journal (GMJ)* 96 (1921) pt. 2, pp.199-200.
8. The Report revealed there were then 201 self-governing burghs in Scotland. 19 of these had a population of less than 1,000 and 108 others with a population of less than 5,000. It was impossible for such units to individually provide the public health services required by the 1920s. The Report suggested replacing these units with larger public health authorities of burghs with over 50,000 population and on county councils of a similar size. Reviewing the 1923 report, the *British Medical*

Journal (BMJ) revealed it had little chance of early success: 'Apart from vested interests, probably the great majority of public health officers will agree that this small number is far better than the present absurd multiplicity, but it seems doubtful whether a bill to give effect to these proposals has much chance to become law, looking to all the influences which would be ranged against it. Perhaps the report, however, may have the effect of leading to some measure of much needed reform'. *BMJ* (1923) pt. 2, 18 Aug. 1923, p.300.

9.   In response to existing local authority vested interests the population unit was set at 20,000 to create 55 new Scottish local authorities.

10.   HOC 9 July 1928, vol. 219 col. (1986).

11.   House of Lords debates (HOL), Viscount Novar , 30 July 1923, vol. 54, col. 1457.

12.   William Adamson MP for West Fife (1910-31), had been the Labour Party's Secretary for Scotland in 1924. He later served as Secretary of State for Scotland 1929-1931.

13.   HOC 23 Mar. 1927, col. 346.

14.   HOC 5 Mar. 1928, vol. 214, col. 898.

15.   Department of Health for Scotland (DHS) Consultative Council on Medical and Allied Services *Report on Hospital Services* (Edinburgh, 1933).

16.   The Scottish Health Services Committee Report became known after its (second) Chairman, nutritionist Edward Provan Cathcart.

17.   Both Edinburgh Royal Colleges (Physicians and Surgeons) strongly supported the key role of the general practitioner in the health services in their evidence to the Cathcart Committee. See DHS *Committee on Scottish Health Services Report*, [Cmd 5208] (1936), pp.152-153.

18.   PRO CAB 24/262 CP (36) 128 Memorandum by Scottish Secretary, Sir Godfrey Collins on the extension of maternal health services in Scotland, 7 May 1936.

19.   DHS *Committee on Scottish Health Services Report*, p.230.

20.   DHS *A National Health Service* [Cmd 6502] (1944), p.72.

21.   For more on the view that government policy is only influenced by agencies when they tell it what it wants to hear, see Keith Dowding *The Civil Service* (1995), p.111.

22.   *Glasgow Medical Journal* (New Ser.) 21 (1943) pt. 1, p.18.

23.   *BMJ* (1945) pt. 1, p.718.

24.   *Summary Report by the Department of Health for Scotland Committee on Scottish Health Services Report for the year ended 30 June 1945* (Edinburgh, 1945), [Cmd 6661], p.15.

25.   DHS *Health and Industrial Efficiency: Scottish Experiments in Social Medicine* (1943) [HMSO].

26.   PRO MH79/526 Memorandum by Thomas Johnston to Cabinet Home Policy Committee 'Prevention and Control of Tuberculosis', Jan. 1942.

27.   *BMJ* (1943) pt. 1, p.789 Report on the DHS pamphlet *Health and Industrial Efficiency.*

28.   PRO Cab 87/81 War Cabinet Inter-Departmental Committee on Social and Allied Services Memoranda Papers file pp.100-129. Memorandum 112 - DHS 'Health of War Workers', 20 July 1942.

29.   War Cabinet Inter-Departmental Committee on Social and Allied Services (Beveridge Report) *Social Insurance and Allied Services* (1942) [Cmd 6404].

30.   PRO MH76/603 DHS Office Committee on the 'Demobilisation' of the Emergency Hospital Scheme - Scotland, 13 Oct. 1943.
31.   The National Health Service (Scotland) Bill was published on 6 Nov. 1946 accompanied by a White Paper (HMSO Edinburgh, 1946) [Cmd 6946].
32.   HOC debates 10 Dec. 1946, vol. 431, col. 1011.

Table 1

Comparative Maternal Mortality Rates (per 1,000 births), 1918-1948

Year	Scotland	Eng&Wales
1918	7	3.8
1919	6.2	4.4
1920	6.2	4.3
1921	6.4	3.9
1922	6.6	3.8
1923	6.4	3.8
1924	5.8	3.9
1925	6.2	4.1
1926	6.4	4.1
1927	6.4	4.1
1928	7	4.4
1929	6.9	4.3
1930	6.9	4.4
1931	5.9	4.1
1932	6.2	4.2
1933	5.9	4.5
1934	6.2	4.6
1935	6.3	4.1
1936	5.6	3.8
1937	4.8	3.3
1938	4.9	3.1
1939	4.4	2.9
1940	4.2	2.7
1941	4.7	2.8
1942	4.1	2.5
1943	3.7	2.3
1944	3	1.9
1945	2.5	1.8
1946	2.2	1.4
1947	2	1.2
1948	1.1	1

Figure 1

Comparative MMR: Scotland and England and Wales, 1918-48

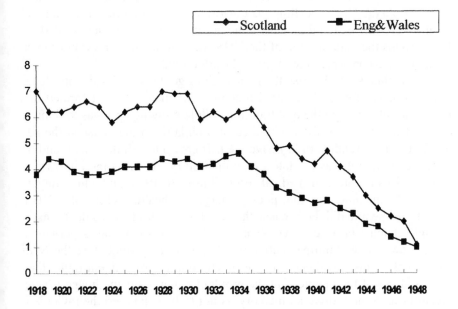

2. Whose Nurse? The Doctor, the District and the NHS

RONA FERGUSON

When first asked to write this paper I thought that I would be able to outline the ways in which the NHS changed the daily work of the district nurse. I expected those I interviewed to have marked the year of the NHS in their memory as that significant year when things changed - but they didn't. They didn't seem to mark the year at all; some couldn't remember which year it was. I was surprised - but why, what did I expect? What is the NHS that it merits 50 year celebrations throughout the country but can also be shrugged off as unmemorable by those who helped to deliver it to us?

As someone far too young to remember 1948 it is easy to think '1948 the introduction of the NHS. Before it there was no universal health care, people died before calling the doctor, and after it there was a National Health Service free to all and everyone got treatment when they needed it.' But perhaps the inauguration of the NHS was not in itself an event or even a singular axis on which the future of health turned.

If this is not the case then where did I get the idea? This introduces a new problem for me because, I imagine, like many others I formed this notion largely through the oral tradition. While growing up I was told many times of my mother's sister who died of diphtheria in the house at the age of 12 because Grandma didn't have the half crown to call the doctor and by the time she did it was too late - a familiar story - but it is the kind which characterises the state of medical services prior to 1948, and which lingers long and romantic, as the public image of health before the NHS. Sometimes people did die because they couldn't afford to see a doctor early enough; it must be true - I've been told the story - but that is perhaps a naive view which is unimaginative in relation to the years before the NHS and reveals a misplaced belief in the functioning of government rather than the resources of the people. But the problem remains - if the image I have, given through the individual memory, is not to be dismissed then why is it that it is now challenged by other individual memories. Why don't the nurses I speak with tell the same story and does the discrepancy devalue the remembered past whatever it tells of?

As the focus of my concern here is to show how the NHS affected the working environment of the district nurse as opposed to the district nursing service and since too the many and various written accounts of the NHS speak little of this I am thrown back to the oral testimonies of those who worked on the district before and after the forties.[1] The difficulty in justifying the value of such testimony is one I will have to return to.

This paper is based on interviews with retired district nurses who worked in Scotland at some time during the period 1940 to 1990.[2] I asked each district nurse about how the NHS affected his or her working life, to be met so often with a puzzled, 'well, it didn't really'. I had to examine my own expectations and focus specifically on what I wanted to know: Surely the new NHS meant no more collecting money by the nurse, people beginning to go directly to the doctor rather than her for advice, surely she saw not only those who had paid for nursing care but a whole new range of patients amongst the poorest in the community? And surely that is worth remembering? Indeed, these are not unusual expectations of the effect of the health service. On the eve of its inauguration The Nursing Times expressed similar optimism for nursing in the community within the new service:

> 'Nurses are fortunate in being a most essential part of the service. Some nurses have been appointed to help in the control and management of it. The majority will, in many people's minds, *be* the service. More nurses will be visiting the homes of the people as health visitors, domestic nurses and midwives. More people will meet the nurse at the clinics, health centres and hospital outpatient departments, and they will judge the service by the personal care and consideration they receive.'[3]

So if nurses didn't readily recall distinct changes directly dependent on the NHS, what did they remember of that time? They remember it only as part of a period of development which brought about many other changes coincident with the effects of the NHS but not fundamental to it; the increase in new drugs and technologies, the move towards more hospital confinements, more married women remaining in active nursing and the growing professionalisation of nursing, to say nothing of reorganisation which has seen informants either bask in the privilege of being a part of it or weep through the personal toll it has taken. All of these have occurred within the overarching context of the NHS and so cannot be separated from it and each has been cited by informants as significant to a perceived change in the nature of district nursing throughout the fifty years since 1948. It is in the face of these changes that the autonomous district nurse of the past, working her district virtually on her own is lamented by the elderly, and the status of skilled professional within the primary care team is achieved by the present day nurse. One particular aspect that is of interest in this paper is the change in working structure over the period and its effect on working relationships.

First I will briefly outline the historical context within which the nurses on the district prior to 1948 understood their work. Home nursing had been practised in some form or other for many years but it was in the late nineteenth century that it became formalised in what is now known as the Queen's Nursing Institute (QNI)[4] which, financed by a gift from Queen Victoria, provided essential training and administration of home nurses and the home nursing service. The late nineteenth century also saw the rise of local district nursing associations, which took on the task of providing home nursing care within their communities. These voluntary committees appointed a nurse, paid her salary, arranged and paid for her accommodation, furnished her house and, in many districts, provided her with transport. In return they expected the nurse to live in the area, nurse the sick, care for the dying, attend confinements where necessary, collect due fees and report to the committee on a regular basis. By the 1920s most areas in Scotland had established such associations with the majority willing to become affiliated to the Queen's Nursing Institute, Scotland (QNIS) Affiliation encouraged associations to employ nurses specifically trained for district work but in times of staff shortages general nurses were appointed. The Queen's Nurse, as the district trained nurses were known, in her navy uniform complete with military style epaulettes, became a visible presence among the community representing a commitment to home nursing care grounded in the strict disciplines of hygiene preached and practised in all Queen's training homes.

The associations operated membership schemes entitling members and their families to free home nursing (with the exception of midwifery, which incurred an extra one off payment).[5] Membership subscriptions were collected door to door by committee members or appointed helpers.

Although the associations employed the nurse, she had three further bodies to account to; the Queen's Nursing Institute of Scotland (QNIS) who supervised district nursing training and practice throughout Scotland, the Medical Officer of Health to whom all her records were sent and who produced an annual report of district nursing services and, to a lesser degree, the district GP who requested all new visits and specified the treatment required. For the nurse, the hierarchy was simple. For the patient, they had someone with a degree of medical knowledge living in the community who was accessible to them. There was not the same distance between the patient and nurse as there was between the patient and the doctor, so, often, people would go to her for advice before bothering the doctor.

'Oh very often, through the night...Is that you nurse, knockin on the window, Who is it? Oh it's me, it's me, oh. Can you come, my mother's fallen out the bed, or somebody's nose is bleeding. Have you been to the doctor? No I didn't like to bother him.'[6]

The district nurse then was frequently the first point of contact for a patient within the system of medical care. Inevitably there were some for whom even small regular payments presented hardship and so a number of people did not participate in the schemes. These patients were often not ignored but attended by the nurse operating at a local level who knew their circumstances. Strictly speaking they could be asked to pay a standard fee. In such cases, it was the duty of the nurse to collect the fee and deposit it with the association at the end of each month and in many cases this is what happened but in many more it seems, the nurse simply ignored the matter of money and either made a case to the committee for them to waive the fee or, in some cases, paid it herself.

'We had to fiddle the books so that, you know, those who needed us are nursed free. And it was quite easy to do a fiddle there, because you took your books to the treasurer, you see, and there was no names, nothing, just X number of deliveries and that. So it was easy enough to cover it ... well, we would keep the records, but it would be a number for the treasurer ... And if we got them to join up, you see, just before hand, it was fine. You had to do that sort of thing.'[7]

But cash was not the only method of payment. Many stories are recalled of a parcel of fish or a rabbit being left at the nurse's doorstep and rural and small town nurses often recall attending tinker folks who were unlikely to pay by any other currency. So this is how people received their nursing care at home prior to the NHS. Yes, they paid for it but, spread over the weeks of the year it was for many, affordable, and for the rest it was generally still available at the discretion of the nurse. It is interesting that the nurses interviewed did not have clear memories of any money they collected nor did they want to linger on that point. This, coupled with their expressed definitions of district nursing, suggests that they did not equate economics and nursing albeit that they worked in a period when health care, including home nursing, was not free. It also highlights the level of discretion nurses employed regarding the general well-being of the patients, with consideration of familial and employment circumstances as well as health matters. This holistic approach was a particular feature of the triple-duty nurse who was general nurse, midwife and health visitor all in one.

> 'It was an ideal situation. And I think, really, an ideal kind of job to have, because we did the child welfare, we did the midwifery, we did the child welfare once we had done our health [visiting], we did it even before we had our health visitor certificate. You did the schools ... So that you knew the whole family from a to z, and they knew you, and you didn't need to ask anybody's history. I mean, you more or less knew everybody and they knew you. But it was a very satisfying way to work. Because you knew that you could do your patients, whatever you wanted to do for them. I think it's a more satisfying way.'[8]

As mentioned above, the hierarchy of authority was relatively simple during this period, but there were differences in the working relationships developed in the three major nursing situations; that of the urban nurse living in a group home; the urban nurse living as an individual nurse; and the rural nurse.

Within these, the main distinction was between the situation of the rural and the city nurse. Where the city nurse tended to separate her work from that of other healthcare professionals such as health visitors and midwives, who were separately employed by the local authority, the rural triple-duty nurse encompassed all three roles. In both areas a house was provided for the nurse in her district first by the local associations and after 1948, by the local authority, but in many urban areas, usually the larger towns and cities, nurses' homes also operated. These housed as many as twenty nurses, including a supervisor who organised domestic arrangements and dealt with incoming requests for nursing care from the GP's. With many district nurses being qualified midwives, nurses based in these homes often shared midwifery duties on a rota basis, allowing some periods of regular hours for each nurse when not on call for confinements. Health visitors were employed directly by local authorities as public health workers under the Medical Officer of Health (MOH) and as such were separate from the district nursing service and were not generally accommodated with the nurses and midwives. However, district nurses and health visitors shared a common function in being essentially community based and indeed shared many patients, specifically the mother and new-born child who would be the case of the district nurse for the first fourteen days after delivery until the health visitor took over. The urban nurse then, when housed with other nurses tended to have ready made social and professional support in her colleagues, who shared the home although she had little contact with the doctors who communicated mainly through the nursing Supervisor. Such nurses worked informally in a team and they tended to be less involved with their patient community.

The urban nurse living independently worked individually. With no supervisor to take calls she had more contact with doctors but found less professional support among nursing colleagues although neighbouring nurses had opportunities to meet up and covered off-duty for each other. Her involvement in the community varied depending on the density of population, the nurse's length of service and whether or not she was also fulfilling the role of midwife.

By contrast, the rural triple-duty nurse fulfilled the role of midwife, health visitor and general nurse in what was often a widespread but sparsely populated area. Often remote from supervisors and even neighbouring districts nurses, she could feel isolated both geographically and professionally. Having a house provided within the district, she became a central figure of her community and was seen by her patients as being on-call twenty four hours a day not just as nurse, but often as confidant and counsellor too. Off-duty and holiday relief was only informally arranged with nurses of nearby districts who, for that period would have to cover both their own and the off-duty nurse's cases. The Association committee was merely administrative and could give no advice on nursing care. Indeed it would have been unprofessional to discuss a patient with them at all unless relevant to a financial matter. Although most GP's are recalled as having been helpful, approachable and cognisant of the nurse's task and ability to do it, some were aloof and ignorant of the nurse's high standard of training, viewing them either as a threat or a handiwoman in uniform. Nurse/doctor relationships tended to be good professional ones with the nurse sometimes sharing the patient's deference to the doctor. Only in a very few cases could they be described as friends.

'No. No. I used to keep the doctors, you know, I would be pleasant, courteous to them, but I never would have lived in a doctor's pocket, you know. Some of the doctors used to say, oh come, we're going out tonight, come out with us. I said, well, I'd have made an excuse or something, no thank you. And locally, you know, if you had seen the nurse go into a house, you know, is she talking about me? You had to think on that side of things. So if you had friends, you would have had friends outwith the district so that they didn't see your car at the door. Because it's terribly important, if the nurse is seen, she's been in the house for an hour. You know, they timed you, how long you'd been in.'[9]

In short, the rural nurse was often locked into her community by having little time off, was more familiar than the doctor and so more frequently called upon for minor complaints In her triple-duty role she was exposed to more information about patients, was privy to more individual confidences relating to health, familial and social circumstances, yet had to straddle the professional demands of her work and her own individual social needs within the same community. The relationships she developed within this context were crucial both to her practice as a community nurse and to her own personal fulfilment. It is not surprising that the rural triple-duty nurse placed much emphasis on these relationships, although prudence dictated that she preserve a degree of social distance to maintain her professionalism.

For many, in retirement, it is the recollection of these relationships which define not only their work as a district nurse but, in many cases, their own lives. District nursing is defined by them in terms of the relationships they formed because, in their experience, these were integral to its function. This attitude reverberates in a minor controversy of the 1960s surrounding the introduction of sterile packs, which was initially viewed as a change set to undermine the nurse/patient relationship. Unlike the small nursing associations of the past, Local Health Boards had the resources to set up central sterile supply services issuing first autoclaved syringes and later other instruments, sterile dressings and so on. Although sometimes viewed as wasteful, the introduction of the sterile pack made a significant impact on the district nurse's working day by removing the need for time consuming home sterilisation of the bake in the biscuit tin variety.[10] Coupled with improved technology, the central sterile supply was a feature of local authority organisation which would not have been possible under the previous system and therefore a direct result of the NHS, although it wasn't until the sixties that it became widespread practice. Then, it sparked debate amongst nurses and, in 1961 became the subject of a survey by the QNI and the main topic of an Institute conference. The principle arguments against it suggested that nurses would require two techniques, one for the sterile pack and another for sterilisation of additional materials in the home, and that they would lose valuable time spent talking to patients through having to collect the supplies. 'When would the nurse have time to say the extra word of comfort and cheer to the patient, and even more important, have time to listen to the patient?'[11]

This time to listen to the patient is recalled as a primary feature of district nursing and the visibility of the nurse meant it was called for in various situations.

> 'I walked in Whitburn; I did a lot of my consultations on my two flat feet. You used to meet people on the streets ... you could deal with a lot of things they wanted to know on the street, yes. These were just people you bumped into, there was something wrong with the family or there was something wrong with them and they would ask you, you know, do you think I should see about this? And I mean sometimes they were quite serious things ... women with a lump in their breast or with abnormal bleeding, or you know something like that. And they would ask you on the street.'[12]

It is this familiarity with the nurse as someone in the community who was not only knowledgeable of medical matters, but approachable and separate from the doctor which was perceived by elderly informants as representing the key conceptual difference between the district nurse before the NHS and until the 1960s, and that of today.

So what impact did the NHS have that may have affected this aspect of the district nurse's work? It has often been reported that with the NHS GP's were inundated with new patients stacking out their surgeries with minor complaints which they would hitherto have dealt with at home, thereby exercising their right to free treatment and indeed the policy of preventive medicine by visiting their doctor before a medical crisis arose. Presumably this took some of the strain off the district nurse as people could then go straight to the doctor without first approaching her, as so often happened in the years before 1948. But the NHS didn't make the doctor instantly more approachable on a personal level and so, where deference to the GP existed, it tended to continue.

> Everybody still went to her when anything was wrong they went to see the nurse ... before they went to see the doctor, an that was after she'd retired ... The doctors took exception to it, they objected to it ... they said

why do they come to you, I said, I don't know why they come to me, I'm
the nearest I suppose ... they didnae want to bother the doctor.[13]

In close communities the nurse was seen as somehow belonging to
the people as a kind of medical mother figure and so they continued to go
to her first before the doctor. But this benign relationship clearly didn't
always prevail as some interpreted their rights within the NHS as
ownership of the medical service and the time of those working within it.

We had only been in this district about six months when the NHS really
erupted to be flagged down by a miner sayin', are you the new nurses,
ye'll hae tae come tae ma hoose, ma wife's needin a bath. I said, well,
what's wrong with yur wife? She's got the flu an that's nae business o
your's, she's needin a bath. I said, well that's really not how we work it, if
your wife's ill certainly we'll nurse her, but doctor decides which patients
need nursing, so see Dr Thwaites and he'll tell us if we come. But he had
now discovered that he was paying us because we were NHS and he was
a worker so he would tell us to come ... the initial impact was that they
were now the bosses, we were there to give a service and they would tell
us...[14]

Furthermore, with more people taking advantage of the new free
service, doctors' caseloads were increasing and within a very short time the
overburdening effect of the NHS on the GP and the home nurse was
evident. In 1950 the Nursing Times reported three main reasons for the
increased demand on the district nurse: the shift from private to public
nursing; the shortage of hospital beds causing patients, especially the
chronic sick or tuberculous, to be ill at home for longer while awaiting
hospital admission, and the early discharge of post-operative and other
acute cases; and the tendency of overworked GP's to rely on home nurses
to do more dressings and injections.

Although in the same year the district nursing service was
described as the most economical section of the NHS,[15] the need to
improve efficiency throughout the medical services was becoming clear.

In the wake of this, clinic work was encouraged and new schemes
formed, notably GP attachment and the Health Centre. Opinions vary as to
the value of each but that they made an impact on working relationships in
the community was almost unanimous amongst those I have interviewed.

From its beginnings in 1948 the NHS had encompassed family
medicine as a crucial issue, with a call to develop Health Centres
throughout the country, but this engendered anxiety in doctors who feared

for their independence. However, there was a recognition of the need to build up an integrated community health policy relying on and expanding on existing community health services such as district nurse and health visitors. Despite this, those who knew this aspect of health care best, that is the nurses working either in hospital or in the community, were not consulted, with Bevan stating, 'if the nurses were to be consulted, why not also the hospital domestics? the radiotherapists? the physiotherapists? and so on'.[16] This in contrast to the position conceded to doctors who obtained a monopoly of legitimacy among the health service providers; a unique position, reflected in the participation of doctors in the running of the NHS.[17] With this the precedent was set for the GP's centrality and superiority in community provision within the NHS. The Health Centre was supposed to ease integration of the local authority health services and the GP's by providing a co-operative interface for professionals linking hospital, family, school and social services together. The social worker, health visitor, district nurse, midwife, chiropodist, physiotherapist, dentist. could all share the resources of the centre to some degree. Teamwork was the key and the team was to be based firmly within the community, accessible to all it served. Although in the proposals, Health Centres were to be a cornerstone of the new all-encompassing health service, the capital investment required was not forthcoming from central government, and there remained much suspicion amongst GP's, still protecting their non-salaried independence. Consequently, it was not until the late sixties that health centres were built in any numbers although Sighthill in Edinburgh did have one of the first four experimental units to be built in the country in 1953. So this major organisational change to affect the work of nurses on the district did not materialise with the coming of the NHS. Doctors still worked from their own practices and nurses still took their cases from them with little or no formal communication. But as local authorities dedicated more clinic buildings for the public health doctors' clinics, the GP's began to encroach on the nurses' territory.

> Of course we got clinics built here and that was a tremendous change, oh we got real clinics buildings that instead of going into the clinic after the school dinners and sweeping up the potatoes off the floor and the chiropodists also used that, I can remember sweeping it up and there would be potato peelings and toenails and then the babies came in... Instead of that we had absolute buildings, but that didn't last very long because the GP's got in ... The GP's used the premises. When the first clinic was built ... it was small right enough but nevertheless it was our

own and that was great and the public health doctor would say 'Now isn't this marvellous, we've got a place of our own and you sit in there and I'll sit in there and the mothers will sit there.' and we could even have little lectures with the mothers you know. But that didn't last because the GP's wanted premises - and when he came into our new clinic of course he brought with him receptionists and suddenly the place was packed and it did cause friction ... you couldn't get room to use as an office... it was wonderful to have these buildings ... we even had fathers coming, it was way ahead ... everything was going well and then the GP's were asking unbeknown to us, could we not be got rid of ... what got me was I had a colleague who had become a Nursing Officer and it really sank me when she said one day, 'was there not a room and kitchen somewhere that we could use'. Now to me that was going back 20 years. The GP's wanted the space.' [18]

In this case the local health authority eventually extended the clinic and the GP's and nurses remained. However, the nurse recounting this, who fought to retain her right to the premises, left district nursing under the strain and took up a full time post as Health Visitor in a neighbouring town.

In the absence of dedicated premises and the promised health centres and in an effort to potentiate the doctor's clinical efficiency,[19] schemes of GP attachment were implemented by urban local authorities. Nurses selected as suitable were attached to particular doctors to help increase the efficiency of medical care and improve the doctors performance. In practical terms this meant that they no longer visited patients within a specific geographical location but only those on the books of the doctor concerned. It was a scheme that had implications for the administrators as well as the nurses on the district:

When the Health Boards took over we were all immediately reassessed ... and if we got a post we became Nursing Officers from that point on ... In Queens as an administrator you [had] still felt very much a part of the whole thing ... the nurse reported to us every day, we knew the patients ... one morning a call came through, this lady very distressed her husband with terminal cancer she'd say Oh I'm sorry but the nurse hasn't come and my husband's in terrible pain, well, we would just immediately pick up a nursing bag jump in a taxi and up to the patient's house and we were used to going round with the nurse so the patients knew the administrators very well and you felt very much a part. From the time I became a Nursing Officer and they started streaming the nurses off to the doctors' surgeries the gap widened and I would say as a Nursing Officer I felt quite isolated, I suffered isolation in that respect.[20]

Despite this, two reports in 1969 and 1971[21] describe the schemes as successful in that patients became familiar with *their doctor's* nurse, the doctor developed a keener awareness of the nurse's skills and workload, and the way was paved for the development of the practice nurse. As communication between doctor and nurse improved this engendered a new appreciation of the nurse's abilities. The nurses began to undertake more clinical work in the surgeries and in effect became a part of the medical service offered by the doctor.

Both these schemes have generated comment among the nurses interviewed as significant factors of change and generally a central base was seen as an advantage to nurse, doctor and patient. In material terms, the purpose built health centres provided a place to store materials, equipment and records, to co-ordinate tasks with colleagues and to initiate group programmes like antenatal clinics, which were time-consuming on an individual basis. It offered the nurse regular contact with doctors (sometimes ten operating from the one health centre) and other health professionals throughout the day. Doctors became more aware of the nurse's high skill level and how this could be utilised. Through delegation to the nurse, the doctor's caseload was significantly reduced in terms of chronic cases, follow-up home visits and, where the nurse held clinical sessions, follow-up and initial cases in the surgery. Patients with minor complaints could often see the nurse quicker than the doctor which led to a more efficient medical service, but while this allowed a diagnostic element into the nurse's work it also reinforced the doctor's medical authority. With an ever growing patient community in the over 65 age group much of the nurse's work for some time had been social bathing, general care and continued care of the chronic sick, conditions which could be handled adequately by State Enrolled Nurses who were now beginning to be employed to take on such visits. This allowed the skilled district nurse freedom to develop clinic work with the GP or attend difficult cases. In the rural setting, despite the demise of triple-duties, this development of the nurse's role in relation to the GP has been viewed as an enhancement of her professional status while the disappearance of the nurse has been mediated by the continued closeness of a small community. In urban areas where these schemes prevailed, the nurse began to move away from the traditional role of the district nurse who was rooted in a geographically defined community and often had to drop some of her patients and travel greater distances to new patients well outside her previous boundary. With closer links as the doctor's assistant, based in the health centre or practice, the district nurse was no longer seen as the nurse of a community of people but was the potentiator of the doctor's clinical efficiency whether in the surgery or patients' homes. The nurse's autonomy was further undermined by an ever-growing team of variously skilled professionals within which patient care was delegated and the service fragmented.

> They're all attached to the Health Centre. There's two Health Centre's in Hawick, and they're attached to that ... and they all work from there. People of my generation we think it isn't all that good. But of course, the people who are doing it think it's better. ... People don't get; they get somebody different every time they come. They don't always get the same person. Whereas in the days when there was a nurse living in the community, everybody knew her. They knew who was coming. They knew, even if they didn't like her. And I think that makes a big difference, whereas they never know who's coming now ... it can be one person one day and one another.[22]

The comment above sums up the reaction of retired district nurses, many now recipients of home care, to the changed system. It may be a view distorted by time, age and the flaws of memory but it nevertheless represents a popular perception. The transition from voluntary to statutory control and the increase in demand for community based nursing has imposed new structures on the organisation of home nursing bridging the gap between the doctor and the nurse. The nurse, now largely invisible is an integral part of the general medical service offered by the doctors either in the surgery or from a centre. To a large extent this has taken the nurse out of the district where she was originally a separate entity with whom people, as patients within that community, could develop a unique relationship.

Notes

1.   This paper is based on oral testimonies collected between 1997 and 1999. Where permission was given, real names have been published; otherwise they have been withheld on request.
2.   A total of 69 interviews were collected as part of a research project instigated by the Queen's Nursing Institute, Scotland with continued funding provided by the Wellcome Trust. Interviews were gathered from retired district nurses who had worked in various locations throughout Scotland including urban, rural and island areas. Recordings of the interviews will be archived in the Royal College of Nursing archive, Edinburgh.

3.   *The Nursing Times* Sat July 3, 1948 Vol.XLIV No.27 p.471.

4.   The Queen's Nursing Institute began in 1887 as the Queen Victoria Jubilee Institute for Nurses gaining a Royal Charter in 1889. In 1925 it changed its name to the Queen's Institute for District Nursing and later became known as the Queen's Nursing Institute (QNI). Throughout this paper it will be referred to as the QNI or QNIS (Queen's Nursing Institute, Scotland).

5.   There were three Schemes for Nursing Services available in 1943. The home nursing Contributory Scheme involving an annual payment of 4s4d at the place of employment to cover the employee and all non-wage earning dependants; the Membership Scheme where the annual payment was 6s and was collected regularly from the member's home, and the subscribing Donor Scheme which entitled domestic staff to free nursing care along with the employer on payment by the employer of 10s per annum. See Annual Report 1943, Queen's Institute of District Nursing, Scottish Branch, QNI Scotland Archive, Edinburgh.

6.   Name of informant withheld by request.

7.   From the testimony of Miss E. Davidson QNIT 21/2 , RCN archive.

8.   Name of informant withheld by request.

9.   From the testimony of Miss E. Davidson QNIT RCN archive.

10.   Before the central sterile supply service nurses sterilised dressings and equipment in patients' homes. See Ferguson, R. 'Recollections of Life 'on the district' in Scotland, 1940-1970' in Bornat, J., Perks, R., Thompson, P. & Walmsley, J. *Oral History, Health and Welfare*, Routledge, (1999), p.153.

11.   *District Nursing* January 1961, No.10, Vol.3, p264.

12.   Name of informant withheld by request.

13.   From the testimony of Miss E Gunn QNIT 10/1, RCN Archive.

14.   From the testimony of Miss J Himsworth QNIT 17/1, RCN Archive.

15.   Address by Dr. Godber at refresher course for HVs in Sept The NHS after two years, in *The Nursing Times*, Nov.18, Vol.46, (1950).

16.   Public Records Office, MH 77/73, Letter from A Bevan to Sir Walter Citrine, the TUCs General Secretary, dated 18 July 1946 quoted in Klein, R. *The Politics of the NHS*, p.21.

17.   Klein, R., *The Politics of the NHS*, p.28.

18.   From the testimony of Miss J Livingstone QNIT 60/1, RCN Archive.

19.   MacGregor, S.W., Heasman, M.A. & Kuenssberg, E.V. *The Evaluation of a Direct Nursing Attachment in a North Edinburgh Practice*, Scottish Home and Health Department, (1971).

20.   From the testimony of Miss E. Gates QNIT 57/2, RCN Archive.

21.   Abel, R A, *Nursing Attachment to General Practice*, Social Services Research Unit Study No.1, HMSO, London 1969. MacGregor, S.W., Heasman, M.A. & Kuenssberg, E.V. *The Evaluation of a Direct Nursing Attachment in a North Edinburgh Practice*, Scottish Home and Health Department, (1971).

22.   From the testimony of Miss C. Campbell QNIT 32/1, RCN Archive.

3. No Wonder Nurses Quit! What the New Health Service meant for Nurses in 1948

SUSAN McGANN

This paper charts the progress of the threatened resignation of over 600 student nurses in London in July 1948. The first part of the paper follows the course of the student nurses' protest and how it was managed by the professional organisations and trade unions. In the second part of the paper the background to the dispute and some of the problems within nursing at the birth of the National Health Service are considered.

The title *No Wonder Nurses Quit!* is taken from an article in the magazine *John Bull,* on 17 July 1948,[1] describing the conditions of student nurses, a familiar list of petty rules, sergeant-major discipline, long hours and poor pay, first recorded in the 1930s and which were still casting a shadow in the 1970s.[2]

John Bull was surprisingly close to the pulse of student nurses' feelings, within three days of this article being published a threatened student nurses' strike hit the front pages of the countries' newspapers. The unrest began on 20 July 1948 when student nurses at St Mary's Hospital, Plaistow, in the East End of London, opened their first pay packets from their new employer the National Health Service. They were shocked to find they were worse off than before, instead of receiving approximately £3 16s 2d, they received £3 3s 4d. Unbeknown to them, they had become liable under the National Insurance Act for contributions amounting to £9 19s 4d per annum, and a compulsory superannuation contribution of approximately £9 0s 0d per annum, a total of just under £19 0s 0d. Previously their deductions had amounted to £4 6s 8d per annum.

They wrote to the Minister of Health, Nye Bevan to the Chairman of their Regional Hospital Board, and to their local MP, pointing out that the additional deductions from their salaries had reduced the net salary to a sum on which it was impossible to exist, and that the nurses in training at St Mary's, Plaistow (approximately seventeen) would have to tender their resignation with effect from 1st August 1948, concluding 'we trust you will see your way clear to amend this matter and thus uphold a distinguished profession'.[3]

The student nurses also sent a letter to over thirty nurses' training schools in England and Wales drawing their attention to the difference in net salaries and informing them of the action they had taken and asking for their support. The following letter was sent to the press:

'With reference to the National Health Scheme, are the public aware that the people most opposed to the scheme are the student nurses. Due to further reductions in an already inadequate salary the student nurses salary will now be, 1st year £3 3s 4d per month, 2nd year £3 19s 0d per month, and 3rd year £4 14s 0d per month. Plus a further reduction of 3s 10d every third month.

Surely since so much consideration has been given to the doctor's salaries a little thought could have been spared for the people, who will make the scheme possible.

Unless something is done the student nurse will cease to exist, not from choice, but necessity.'[4]

The Ministry of Health responded by announcing that the Nurses' Salaries Committee (Rushcliffe Committee) had recommended that student nurses should have an additional £15 0s 0d per annum, and that this had been accepted and was to come into immediate effect. This rise still left the student nurses poorer by some £3 0s 0d per annum on their pre-July salary and this badly timed announcement of an already agreed plan merely roused their anger further.

The threatened resignations of the student nurses was well covered by the press, as the National Health Service was news at the time. The student nurses at St Mary's called a meeting for 9.30 p.m. on 22 July. The hospital was reported to be in an uproar with press reporters flocking in. Nurses from supporting hospitals were invited to the meeting. In all approximately six hundred student nurses from hospitals in the east end of London, including Whipps Cross Hospital, the Prince of Wales's Hospital, Bethnal Green Hospital, and East Ham Memorial Hospital, had threatened to resign. Telegrams and telephone messages were received from all over England and one from Scotland supporting the claims and expressing readiness to follow the lead of the St Mary's nurses.

Two of the sisters at St Mary's offered to conduct the meeting and it was agreed to seek a meeting with representatives of the Royal College of Nursing. At this meeting, which took place the next morning, the students wanted to discuss not just salaries but also hours of duty, examination fees, holidays, the recent increase in the deductions in pay, and reduced travel rates. During this meeting two members of the Regional Hospital Board were present and afterwards met the students and asked them to withdraw their resignations, which they did.

An open meeting for student nurses was held at 9.30 p.m. on 23 July at the Royal College of Nursing. The meeting was well covered by the press which described the event in the following terms: 'More than 1000 student nurses from all over London and the Home Counties besieged the Royal College of Nursing last night to demand more pay ... Although many of the nurses did not get off duty until less than an hour before the meeting was due to begin, they forfeited their suppers and trekked across London by bus, tube, taxi, car and on foot.'[5]

After the meeting a press statement from the Royal College of Nursing stated that the protesting students were now in consultation with the College and that the matter would be referred to the new negotiating machinery set up under the National Health Service, the Whitley Council for Nurses and Midwives. The statement outlined the College's stand on the status of student nurses,

> 'In the opinion of the College emphasis in future must be placed on her status as a student rather than as an employee of the hospital. The College has always maintained that if the nurse in training is to be recognised as a genuine student of nursing her remuneration during training should take the form of educational grants and adequate maintenance allowances (a policy which has the whole-hearted support of the College Student Nurses' Association) rather than salary or wages as an employee.'[6]

Some of the protesting student nurses were members of trade unions and the biggest unions involved, the Confederation of Health Service Employees (COHSE) and the National Union of Public Employees (NUPE), also held meetings with the students. The message from all these organisations was to stay at work and they would bring the matter before the Whitley Council.

The medical press was also interested in the student nurses plight and the Lancet observed that 'It is stimulating to find nurses - who usually seem too busy or too tired for polemics - taking an active line for once.

Many will sympathise with their protest, especially since - in the best traditions of their profession - they are prepared to stay at work for a time after Aug 1st in order to give the hospitals a chance of getting new staff.' The Lancet concluded that a fresh study of the pay of student nurses was urgently needed and that it was unfortunate that their claims had been neglected and so mismanaged that they had been driven to forcible protest.[7]

The climax of the dispute was a public march from Trafalgar Square to Hyde Park organised by COHSE on 15 Aug 1948. A member of the staff of the Royal College of Nursing attended the demonstration in Hyde Park and in a written report described the proceedings,

> ... the nurses were in the main a rag-tag and bob-tail crowd, obviously mental nurses and assistant nurses, with a large number of male nurses, in uniform, in mufti, hats on, hats off, hair blowing, coats dangling from arms, bare legged, and all slumicking along anyhow.
>
> ... Speakers abused the College and its activities on the Rushcliffe Committee; nurses would never get a square deal while 'that matron-ridden institution dominated the Whitley Council'; it had refused to support the claims made by the trade unions and had been instrumental in downgrading the claims which the trade unions had wanted to forward for the student nurses ...
>
> ... My own personal opinion is that the immediate issue is COHSE endeavouring to oust the College from any negotiating body by large increases of membership, and that COHSE is being used along with the nursing profession by a far more significant force, as a political weapon.[8]

The editor of the Nursing Times also attended the demonstration and filed the following report,

> At the COHSE meeting in Hyde Park on Sunday, August 15, numerous trade union officials spoke at length about the need for nurses to join a union to get improvements.... Around us were middle aged and elderly pipe-smoking trade unionists, with a few amused State Registered Nurses. The meeting was orderly and dull while long historical reports were given ... The resolution calling on the Whitley Council to give £5 0s 0d per week was passed ... The meeting degenerated into a hospital porter and a few trades unionists talking about beetles and ants in the porter's hospital ... The impression was that there is not complete co-ordination and good feeling between the nurse members and the officials of the union.[9]

The meeting of the relevant committee of the Whitley Council to consider the student nurses' pay claim took place on 13 August 1948 and it was agreed that an increase was justified by the rise in the cost of living. Accordingly the Staff Side of the Nurses and Midwives Whitley Council made a case for increased pay and emoluments which would leave the student nurse with not less than £2 0s 0d a week in her pocket after all statutory deductions had been made. At the end of 1948 the Whitley Council agreed to an increase in student nurses' pay, amounting to a rise of £5 0s 0d a week or £8 0s 0d monthly.

It was further agreed that nurses-in-training were student nurses and they should be paid a training allowance. The training allowance was raised to £200 per annum. The whole allowance was subject to insurance and superannuation deductions, and consequently the student nurse did not become a true student with the usual student privileges and contacts.[10]

The Political Context

The story about poorly paid nurses being victimised by their employers is always popular with the press and the public but in July 1948 it was extremely topical. Nobody missed the contrast between the high handed treatment of the nurses and the conciliatory treatment of the doctors by the government. The wider political context was the end of a decade in which there had been an unprecedented number of studies of the nursing workforce. At the same time, the Ministry of Health was involved in discussions about the reform of the hospital services and the shape of post-war health services.

Since 1939 staff of the Ministry had been involved in setting up enquiries on nurses' salaries, nurse recruitment, in drafting legislation on the assistant nurse, and in the wartime proceedings of two advisory councils on nursing. The first of these government enquiries was the Interdepartmental Committee on the Nursing Services (Ministry of Health and Board of Education), chaired by the Earl of Athlone, and appointed in 1937 to inquire into the present arrangements concerning the recruitment, training, registration and terms and conditions of service of persons engaged in nursing the sick. The committee published an interim report in 1938 and, despite the start of the Second World War, the Ministry was put under considerable pressure by the nursing organisations to act on some of the more urgent recommendations.

The most urgent was the recommendation that nurses' salaries and pensions should be dealt with on a national basis. The Ministry had also received requests from the employers to set up some central mechanism to standardise salaries for nurses.[11] The result was the appointment by the Minister of Health of the Nurses' Salaries Committee under the chairmanship of Lord Rushcliffe, in October 1941, to negotiate national salary scales for the nursing profession. A similar committee was appointed in Scotland under the chairmanship of Prof. Taylor.

The Committees were a necessary step to harmonise the pay and conditions of service of nurses before a National Health Service structure could be introduced. They consisted of two panels representing the employers and the nurses. The government wanted the committees to deal with just salaries, but the nurses' organisations and unions insisted that salaries could not be considered without including pensions, hours and conditions and subsequently the terms of reference were widened to include these.

Committees, Rushcliffe and Taylor, recommended raising and standardising salary scales. To meet the substantial costs of the salary awards grants were to be made available by the Treasury thus involving the government to a large extent in the cost of the country's nursing service.[12] The Rushcliffe committee continued to sit right up until the hand over to the National Health Service when it was replaced by the Nurses and Midwives Whitley Council. One of the last subjects that the Rushcliffe Committee considered was the issue of student nurses' pay. However the two sides were unable to agree. The employers side was not prepared to concede more than a £15 0s 0d a year rise which the staff side felt unable to accept.[13]

Both sides refused to compromise. The staff side considered taking action under the Conditions of Employment and National Arbitration Order 1940, but were advised by the Ministry of Labour that the circumstances of the case did not constitute a trade dispute. Lord Rushcliffe himself went to the Ministry, but they would not intervene and advised the committee to leave the matter over for the Whitley Council to consider. However, in June 1948 it was agreed that the £15 0s 0d increase per annum would be paid as an interim measure, unfortunately the Ministry forgot to inform the student nurses about this payment.[14] Although the Ministry of Health provided a secretary to the committee, it was not a part of his function to lay down the parameters of negotiation unlike in the Committee's successor the Whitley Council where the Department of Health and Ministry of Labour were directly represented on the management side and government ministers prescribed the limits within which the negotiations should take place.

A second controversial subject that involved the Ministry at this time was the position of assistant nurses. The shortage of trained nurses throughout the 1920s and 1930s had created a situation in which a large part of the nursing workforce was now composed of assistant nurses who had no formal training or registration. The Nurses Registration Acts in 1919 had made no provision for a second grade of nurse. In 1942 the Ministry of Health bowed to pressure from the nurses' professional organisations and the employers of nurses and prepared legislation to regularise the status of the assistant nurse. The Nurses' Act, 1943, empowered the General Nursing Council, the statutory body, to establish a Roll for Assistant Nurses.

The demands of the war forced the government to become involved in the recruitment and distribution of the nursing workforce. The Emergency Medical Service was set up by the Ministry to ensure a co-ordinated service was available across the country to deal with military and civilian casualties. The Ministry of Health was responsible for ensuring the availability of staff to care for these casualties, and set up the Civil Nursing Reserve (CNR) and the Civil Nursing Reserve Advisory Council, in April 1940. As part of the work involved in managing the Emergency Medical Service, the Ministry undertook regular surveys of hospitals, collecting information on the available nursing workforce and the level of shortages. As a result the Ministry was aware of nurse staffing levels and of regional variations in the nursing services.[15]

In February 1942, the Ministry of Labour and National Service set up the National Advisory Council to consider the recruitment and distribution of nurses and midwives. This council, like the Nurses' Salaries Committees, was representative of the various groups of employers and employees. It met quarterly during the war and carried out a survey of 'nurse power', recruitment programmes and propaganda through the press, posters, broadcasts and films.[16]

Before the appointment of the Nurses' Salaries Committee in October 1941, the Royal College of Nursing appointed a working party to consider firstly, how the recommendations of the Inter-departmental Committee on Nursing Services [Athlone] could be implemented and, secondly, the future of the nursing services in the post-war health services. Known as the Nursing Reconstruction Committee and under the chairmanship of Lord Horder, the committee comprised twenty three representatives from the College and twenty five from kindred associations, including the British Medical Association, King Edward's Hospital Fund for London, the Society of Medical Officers of Health, Nuffield Provincial Hospitals Trust, the Trades Union Congress and the British Hospitals Association.

The Horder Committee produced its first report in 1942 on the Assistant Nurse, and a combined report on Education and Training, and Recruitment, in 1943. A final report on the Social and Economic Conditions of the Nurse was published in 1949. Although it is considered that the Horder reports contributed little of substance to the reconstruction of nursing during wartime[17] it may be that the committee's vision that 'nursing is not merely an item in the nation's medical service, but a profession parallel to that of medicine, occupying an appointed and increasingly important place in the national plan for health' was unpalatable to the Ministry at the time and it preferred to appoint its own committees.[18]

The last report on the nursing profession before the introduction of the National Health Service was the Working Party on the Recruitment and Training of Nurses, appointed by the Minister of Health in 1946, under the chairmanship of Sir Robert Wood. This working party was asked to assess the nursing workforce required for the future health service and make recommendations as to how such a workforce could best be recruited, trained and deployed.

The working party's recommendations, contained in a majority report, were published in 1947, months before the introduction of the National Health Service. At this stage it was too late to change the composition of the nursing workforce that the new health service would inherit. All the problems associated with nursing in the inter-war years, shortages, wastage, poor working conditions, inadequate salaries, out of date training, were carried over into the second half of the twentieth century.

The Professional Context

This story of the threatened resignations of 600 student nurses, the trade union led demonstration in Hyde Park, and the Ministry forgetting to announce the £15 0s 0d per annum rise, highlights some of the problems within nursing at this time. The Ministry of Health was attempting to form a national nursing service out of many diverse groups. Before 1948 nurses worked for many different employers, voluntary hospitals, municipal hospitals, local authority services, domiciliary nursing and a wide variety of private and voluntary organisations. Within these groups there were different traditions and loyalties dating back to their distinct origins in the nineteenth century.

The two dominant traditions were the professional and the trade union movements. The former dated back to the 1880s and the beginning of the campaign for state registration for nurses. The founders of that campaign believed that nursing could be a profession for intelligent women and this vision was taken up by subsequent organisations including the (Royal) College of Nursing when it was founded in 1916.[19] The introduction of state registration for nurses in 1919 did not pull the different groups together. On the contrary the Nurses Registration Acts (England and Wales, Scotland, and Ireland) by establishing national Registers for Nurses with six different parts - general trained nurses, male nurses, mental nurses, sick children's nurses, fever nurses and nurses for the mentally handicapped - deepened the divisions in the nursing workforce.

Because of the professional threat to trained nurses posed by the VAD's in 1916, membership of the College of Nursing was restricted to female nurses with three years general training. Consequently, in the 1920s, 1930s and 1940s the membership and staff of the College were drawn from the General Part of the Nurses' Registers and this group regarded themselves as the leaders of the professional movement in nursing. While many fever nurses and sick children's nurses were also qualified and registered as general nurses, and therefore eligible to join the College, there was very little cross over between nurses qualified in the mental health fields and general nursing.

Traditionally men had been employed as attendants in mental health institutions and this had led to the development of a strong male, trade union culture in mental health nursing. Although the Registration Acts had included parts on the Register for mental nurses and mental handicap nurses, mental health nurses did not identify with the General Nursing Council (GNC), the statutory body, and by 1938 the vast majority of them still took the examination of the Royal Medico-Psychological Association, founded in the nineteenth century, and did not take the state examination or register with the GNC.[20]

This professional divide was underlined by an educational distinction. The nurse training schools attached to the prestigious teaching hospitals could take their pick of the recruits, and they were more likely to select the better educated, forcing the students with lower educational qualifications into the supplementary fields of nursing. They were also more likely to select girls from middle class backgrounds thus creating a class or social divide between the different types of hospital training schools.

For many years the professional organisations and the trade unions which represented nurses had been at odds about whether student nurses were students or employees. The professional organisations argued that they were students and that their pay should not be regarded as a salary. On the other hand the trade unions regarded them as employees and were more concerned about their working conditions than their professional development and education.

The trade unions were concerned with practical issues, with student nurses as part of the labour force the low pay they received had the effect of holding down the wages of auxiliaries, and there was the old problem of the low pay of women holding back the pay of men. Both sides had a vested interest in recruitment: if the student nurses became 'students' they would not be eligible for union membership; but if they remained 'employees' then the Student Nurses' Association of the Royal College of Nursing was not a negotiating body and pressure could be put on them to join a union.

Although student nurses were not eligible to join the College until they had qualified, the College had founded a Student Nurses' Association (SNA) in 1925 and all its professional statements supported the objective that nurses in training should be treated as students. In a Memorandum on Student Nurses' Salaries and Status, issued in July 1948, the SNA stated,

> In the opinion of the College ... student status for the nurse in training is essential if wastage is to be reduced and the maximum economy of nurse power ensured. Instead of a salary she would receive allowances ... sufficient to cover the cost of board and lodging and such reasonable personal expenses as any student must incur, and which the present student of nursing is quite unable to meet without help.
>
> The Central Representative Council of the SNA recommend therefore a completely new approach to their method of remuneration. Instead of receiving emoluments in kind the student nurse should henceforth be paid a gross salary on which she would be liable for income tax, out of which she would pay the hospital for the costs of residence ... Gross salary of £275 0s 0d per annum, rising to £300 per annum, should be used as a bargaining figure. The advance on present rates appears considerable. In effect it would only ensure a reasonable independence to the careful

nurse, but its effect on the profession as a whole would be altogether salutary.[21]

By the end of 1948, 10,374 student nurses had enrolled in the SNA, over 3,000 more than in any previous year, bringing the total membership to 19,000.[22] These figures would seem to indicate that the majority of student nurses in 1948 considered membership of the SNA of the Royal College of Nursing was in their long term professional interests. The argument for student status was accepted by the Athlone, Rushcliffe and Wood committees but the recommended minimum salaries were ignored by nurses' employers.

Because nursing required so many thousands of recruits each year, and because the minimum educational requirement for entry was low (in 1939 it was dropped completely), recruits into nursing were not coming from the economic background of other students.[23] By 1948 the majority of the recruits were not able to get support from their families during training. Consequently, they relied on their monthly pay packet to survive and it was generally agreed that one could not survive on what a student nurse was 'paid'.

This problem was considered at length in an article in the Lancet, 7 Aug 1948. The article referred back to the Lancet of February 1947 which had outlined the budget for a student nurse receiving £55 0s 0d per annum; £20 0s 0d for essential clothing other than uniform (including underwear, stockings, shoes and shoe repairs, as well as outdoor clothes); £25 0s 0d for expenses when off duty, including fares and modest entertainment; £5-£10 0s 0d for insurance and superannuation; £5 0s 0d for petty items such as cigarettes, tooth-paste, small repairs, Christmas presents, hairdressing, and textbooks. This narrow budget had become even more stringent in the last twelve months as all these items have risen in cost,

> 'In short, to meet all their expenses student nurses must have some help from home: and many of them inevitably come from homes where the parents feel that the grown child should be a contributor, not an expense.'[24]

At the time of the protest, July 1948, all the parties concerned – the Ministry of Health, the hospital managers, the Royal College of Nursing and the trade unions - were aware that there was a problem with student nurses' pay. However, as we have seen, they had been unable to reach agreement through discussions at the Rushcliffe Committee and had been advised by the Ministry to let the subject 'lie on the table' until the Whitley Council negotiating machinery came into operation.

Once the student nurses protested, all agreed that their salaries were unacceptable. The Royal College of Nursing, as the largest of the professional organisations, was the whipping boy for much of the establishment's uneasiness. The following editorial from The Medical Press, was titled *None So Blind...!*

Nelson, in his later career at least, had one great advantage over his fellow men; he had a blind eye to which he could clasp his telescope. The ordinary, intelligent, fully-sighted human being has to indulge in the most fantastic contortions if he is deliberately to avoid seeing what is plainly before his nose. Some months ago we suggested that of all the things which interfere with the recruitment of nurses, one of the most obvious was the smallness of the student nurses' salary. We claimed no special virtue for our perception of this. On the contrary, we implied that it was a fact so plain that there was little excuse for its neglect. It is, therefore, with considerable interest that we have watched for signs that others were also perceiving it.

Instead, we have had to content ourselves with the diverting spectacle of numerous attempts to dodge the issue. Most ingenuous of these was the suggestion by one body of elderly statesmen within the nursing profession that the payment of student nurses was wrong in principle and that the way out of all our troubles was to emphasise the student status of the junior nurse by asking her to pay fees for her training. This is undoubtedly an outstanding instance of the acceptance of the principle that it is more blessed to give than to receive; the altruism of its originators was truly magnificent!

... It has to be argued that if nurses were really dissatisfied they would protest. We suspect that many of them find that the easiest way to protest is to leave the job. It needs more courage and resolution than one can fairly expect of a girl of eighteen to try to organise a collective protest in the authoritarian atmosphere of a hospital. [25]

Conclusion

Having considered the protest of July 1948 and the events leading up to it two questions stand out; first, why were the representatives of the employers on the Rushcliffe committee so uncompromising in their attitude to the staff side's case for a cost of living rise for the student nurses? And second, after many years of poor pay why was this incident the one which tipped the balance for the student nurses at St Mary's Hospital Plaistow?

In considering the first question, it is difficult to understand why the employers expected student nurses to take an unannounced pay cut. Once the protest started and student nurses' salaries were exposed to the public and the media, nobody could defend their meagreness. On top of this, the employers knew by 1948 that they would no longer be responsible for student nurses' salaries under the National Health Service. Given that the Treasury had been paying a proportion of nurses' salaries since 1943 and that the Ministry of Health advised the Rushcliffe committee to let the matter lie on the table until the Whitley Council took over, it seems likely that the Government did not want the student nurses to get a rise in excess of £15 0s 0d per annum. This would fit into the context of a government that was trying to control the already escalating costs of the new health service.[26]

There is no doubt that despite all the information that various government departments had collected on nurses, their pay and conditions, wastage and recruitment during the decade, the Ministry seriously under-estimated the urgency of the student nurses' case. Although several groups had pointed out that the success of the National Health Service would 'depend on the quantity and quality of nurses who are an integral part of the health team',[27] it would seem that to the Ministry the contribution of nurses was considered at a manpower level.

The second question is equally difficult to answer, who or what gave the student nurses at St Mary's the courage to challenge the government, the nursing establishment and the hospital authorities? There was little history of radicalism among student nurses and, as The Medical Press observed, the authoritarian atmosphere of a hospital was not a good breeding ground for revolutionaries. One of the reports, quoted above, by an RCN officer who attended the Hyde Park demonstration referred to the possibility that the student nurses were being used by a left wing group and she picked up a paper at Hyde Park titled 'Florence's Lamp becomes Torch of Freedom'. This paper concludes,

> 'Fellow nurses – the Royal College is seeking to divide us, saying that, as nurses, we are professionals and should not be united in a union. On the other hand, fat-salaried Union Officials are being forced to take action on our behalf. We have no confidence in either of these sets of officials.'[28]

While some nurses were active in left wing politics, this activity had peaked in the 1930s with the publication of Trades Union Congress' Charter for the Nursing Profession and the Socialist Medical Association's Memorandum on Nursing Services.[29] In 1948 the trade unions were as surprised as the professional organisations when the protest erupted and each attempted to exploit the proceedings to their own advantage.

It seems more likely that the 1948 protest was a spontaneous reaction on the part of the student nurses at St Mary's. The East End of London has a proud tradition of radical action and the high-handed treatment by the Ministry of Health, against a background of generous salary increases for doctors, was too great a provocation.

This chapter has looked at one aspect of the introduction of the new health service, student nurses' pay, where there was an immediate effect on the lowest level of the profession. The structure of the new health service would have a profound impact on all aspects of nursing but this was not apparent in 1948.[30]

Notes

1.   RCN 17/2/41, Royal College of Nursing Archives.
2.   The Lancet Commission on Nursing, Report, London 1932; Report of the Committee on Nursing, HMSO (1972).
3.   RCN 17/2/41.
4.   RCN 17/2/41.
5.   Daily Graphic 24 July 1948, RCN17/2/41.
6.   RCN 17/2/41.
7.   The Lancet 7 Aug 1948.
8.   RCN 17/2/41.
9.   RCN 17/2/41.
10. RCN 17/2/41.
11. E. J. C. Scott, 'The Influence of the staff of the Ministry of Health on policies for nursing 1919-1968' (London School of Economics and Political Science, Ph.D. thesis, 1994), p. 123.
12. A.M. Rafferty, *The Politics of Nursing Knowledge* (London, 1996), p.169.
13. RCN 17/2/41.
14. RCN 17/2/41.
15. E. J. C. Scott, 'The Influence of the staff of the Ministry of Health on policies for nursing 1919-1968' (London School of Economics and Political Science, Ph.D. thesis, 1994), p. 135.
16. The Royal College of Nursing, *Nursing Reconstruction Committee*, Report section III, Recruitment, p.75, par. 60.
17. A.M. Rafferty, *The Politics of Nursing Knowledge* (London, 1996), p.172, and E. J. C. Scott, 'The Influence of the staff of the Ministry of Health on policies for

nursing 1919-1968' (London School of Economics and Political Science, Ph.D. thesis, 1994), pp.188-190.

18.   The Royal College of Nursing, *Nursing Reconstruction Committee*, Report section II, Education and Training, p.11, par.13.

19.   S. McGann, The Battle of the Nurses (London, 1992), pp.160-189.

20.   The Royal College of Nursing, *Nursing Reconstruction Committee*, Report section II, p.26, par. 65, and footnote.

21.   RCN 17/2/41.

22.   Royal College of Nursing, Annual Report, (1948).

23.   R. White, The effects of the NHS on the nursing profession 1948-1969 (London 1985), pp.89-119.

24.   The *Lancet*, 7 Aug. 1948, The Pay of a Student Nurse.

25.   RCN 17/2/41, The Medical Press, 18 Aug 1948, Editorial.

26.   C. Webster, The Health Services Since the War, Vol. I, Problems of Health Care, The National Health Service Before 1957 (London, 1988), pp.133-134.

27.   The Socialist Medical Association and the British Medical Association quoted in E. J. C. Scott, 'The Influence of the staff of the Ministry of Health on policies for nursing 1919-1968' (London School of Economics and Political Science, Ph.D. thesis, 1994), p136.

28.   RCN 17/2/41.

29.   C. Nolan, *A Bride for St Thomas* (London, 1970), pp.125-158; A.M. Rafferty, *The Politics of Nursing Knowledge* (London, 1996), p. 158; B. Abel-Smith, *A History of the Nursing Profession* (London, 1960), pp.142-147.

30.   R. White, The Effects of the NHS on the Nursing Profession 1948-1969 (London, 1985).

4. Speaking in a Different Voice? Devolution and Nursing

FIONA O'NEILL

The creation of the National Health Service had an important unifying impact on nursing. The implementation of the Nurses' Registration Act after the First World War had imposed some degree of order and uniformity on the emerging profession. However, the limitations of the Act, coupled with the fragmented nature of health care provision between the wars, meant that nursing continued to be a diverse and highly variable occupation. Registered nurses from different parts of the country working in vastly different hospital and community settings often had little in common apart from their certificate of registration.[1] This situation was to change after 1948 and as nursing took its place within the NHS there followed an inevitable process of change and accommodation to the challenges imposed by the new national organisation and structure.

Over fifty years on and the introduction of political devolution to Scotland, Wales and Northern Ireland once again raises the prospect of a more diverse and variable health service. This paper will make a critical assessment of the implications of Scottish devolution for nursing in the context of the wider development of the NHS. Health is one of the key areas of responsibility for the Scottish Parliament. There are high expectations of what may be achieved in terms of providing a new focus and impetus to health policy and heath care in Scotland. In particular there is hope that more can now be done to develop a service that is more equipped to address the specific healthcare needs of the Scottish people.[2] Leading Scottish nurses have been keen to embrace the opportunities presented by the end of the old order and argue that they are well prepared to take an active role in a revitalised policy community.[3] In addition leading actors in the Scottish health policy community have signalled their support for nurses and nursing. Susan Deacon the Scottish Health Minister has spoken of her commitment to enhance the scope, responsibilities and opportunities for nurses in Scotland at the centre of a patient-centred approach to care.[4] A number of new initiatives are already in place aimed at expanding the role of the nurse in the Scottish NHS.[5]

Nurses may justifiably feel that devolution, when placed in the developing regional agenda and support for increased autonomy within the English regions, holds the potential for all nurses to assume a more influential role in the policy process. In this view a decentralised system, more sympathetic to the concerns and expertise of nurses, could provide an easier climate for nursing leaders to forward their own visions of health and healthcare than the overly centralised and medically dominated pre-devolution NHS.

However, devolution and the prospect of a process of increased divergence between health services raises a number of challenging and interesting questions about the future of nursing not only within Scotland, but also in relation to the United Kingdom as a whole. Could devolution contribute to a process of fragmentation within nursing? This may be a particularly pertinent point in view of the rather fragile unity of the profession. Nursing has long been noted for its divisions and difficulties in finding ways of incorporating the diversity of nursing into effective and pluralistic representative structures. Furthermore, how likely is it that nurses working in Scotland will face a substantially different policy agenda to the one facing nurses elsewhere in Britain? Perhaps most importantly in the context of this paper, is the matter of how nursing leaders in the UK should react to the developing agenda in the post devolution NHS.

The answer to such thorny questions lies to some degree in the likelihood or otherwise of Scotland developing a health care system that is distinctive enough to produce the kind of tensions that could lead to pressures for increased diversity within the existing unitary arrangements that govern nursing. It must be remembered that nursing has developed its modern identity within a national system that has always had separate administrative arrangements in the four countries of the United Kingdom. Health policy in Scotland may have often mirrored or followed arrangements in England, but there have been important differences. A good recent example of this in relation to nursing is the non-adoption of the consortia mechanism for the commissioning of nurse education in Scotland. As a result of Working Paper 10, that was part of the Thatcher Government's Working for Patients reform of the NHS, new arrangements for purchasing nurse education from provider institutions in higher education was implemented in England. Consortia comprising groups of local representatives from health care employers became responsible for the direct purchasing of nurse education in a bid to increase employer control of nurse education and also to introduce an element of competition into the system. These arrangements have not been followed in Scotland where the Scottish NHS Management Executive is responsible for both workforce planning and educational contracting with nurse education institutions.[6] Other significant areas of difference relate to the policy environment in Scotland in comparison with England. What has been described as a policy village within the Scottish NHS means that nursing leaders are more fully integrated into key professional and administrative networks. In effect nurses in Scotland work within a more contained and accessible system, that contrasts to the more complex and highly politicised health policy networks in England.[7] Moreover, in view of the differences that already exist within the two systems, the added dimension of political devolution may logically be expected to lead to a greater divergence. As one health service manager commented: devolution doesn't mean anything unless you do things differently - otherwise why have it? [8]

However, while it is clearly a perilous undertaking to make any predictions about the extent or otherwise of future divergence, there are sound reasons why the NHS may continue to have a very significant national focus at least in the foreseeable future. Now, as in the past, nursing leaders need to find effective strategies with which to engage with the intensely politicised health policy arena at all levels of the NHS, from the local, to the central and increasingly the European level. Health care systems across Europe and elsewhere in an increasingly, globalised world, face similar pressures of ageing populations, technological advance, raised expectations and an expanded notion of what can and should be provided. These pressures have to be also set against a background of anxieties about rising public expenditure and a desire to contain rising healthcare costs. Health policy is now characterised by an almost constant climate of change and crisis. Change affects not only the administrative and political arrangements which determine how health care is delivered but it also has implications in terms of the constant expansion of the possibilities of what a health care system can offer to citizens. At the heart of this issue is the important question of public expectations in relation to health care provision. British people may grudgingly accept that certain treatments and services are more freely available in other European health care systems but are likely to be less sanguine about significant variations in service provision within the UK. The peculiarities of the NHS and the continued adherence, at least on a rhetorical level, to the founding principles based on the principle of comprehensiveness and national provision of services makes the prospect of a more radical divergence even more unlikely. Lastly, the rather myopic view of the impact of developments within the European Union (EU) that prevails in this country should not obscure the already substantial influence that Europe has on policy developments in health and health care here. There are already significant pressures for a degree of convergence or harmonisation within areas such as pre and post registration nurse education designed to make it easier for nurses to move around the EU to work. The European agenda also extends much wider than a concern with the free movement of labour. A commitment to public health and prevention and initiatives such as the Europe against Cancer and Europe against Aids programmes have had an impact. There are now a number of successful and influential organisations that unite nurses across Europe.[9] At the same time European inspired legislation in relation to the employment of other health service personnel, notably the regulation of junior doctor's hours has already contributed to the recent expansion in the role of the nurse. These are trends that in many ways run contrary to the current of devolution and the prospect of increased diversity that it raises.

In sum a case can be made that now as in the past the fortunes of nursing are implicitly tied to the wider political, social and economic context in which the formal health care system is located. In this bigger picture, devolution is just one amongst many challenges that nurses and nursing face in the current climate of change and uncertainty about the long term future of the NHS. Although it is undeniable that devolution adds a significant dimension to nursing in the NHS and also opens up important new channels of influence that nurses can to use to strengthen their voice in local policy making. At the same time, many of the most vital and pressing issues facing policy makers, professionals and the general public alike, including those relating to the role of the nurse, are most likely to continue to be experienced as primarily national issues. Issues such as the shifting boundaries between health professionals, the difficulties in relation to recruitment and retention in nursing, and the associated debate about the preparation needed to be an effective nurse, demands a nationally led and co-ordinated response in order to maximise effectiveness.

Nursing history is often presented as one of thwarted aspiration, with nurses denied the opportunity of advancing their profession by the more powerful medical profession, all in the context of the structural inequalities that constrain a predominantly female workforce.[10] However, while there have been constraints, there have also been opportunities. Now, as in the past, there are gains to be had from keeping a strong focus on improving the effectiveness of their national representative organisations and finding ways to develop more effective strategies with which to capitalise on the current climate of change. In this view any tendency towards fragmentation that devolution may set in motion may best be resisted if the nursing voice is to be heard at its loudest at the most strategic levels of the service.

Nursing and the Foundation of the NHS

The provision of nursing services presented a serious problem as the plans for the new National Health Service neared completion. Fears about both the quantity and the quality of nurses available to staff the new service were widely seen to threaten the potential for success. Nursing shortages had become a matter of increasing concern during the 1930s. As the employment possibilities available to young women slowly began to widen there was concern about how nursing could be made a more attractive career option. The expanding commercial sector began to offer women, who might otherwise have been attracted to nursing, the prospect of more freedom and independence as clerks, typists and shop assistants. There was much discussion of how to attract the town girl into nursing.[11] The various reports and enquiries set up to look at nursing at this time focused on a number of different aspects connected with the training, conditions of service and role of the nurse in the developing hospital service. It was noted that the demand for nurses was rapidly increasing as technical advance and developments in medical expertise helped to fuel the expansion of hospital provision. Attention was also focused on the organisation and structure of nursing. The Report of the Lancet Commission in 1932 was the first in a number of stringent critiques of some of the dominant practices and philosophies within nursing. Critics argued that nursing remained insular and old-fashioned. A strict and hierarchical organisational structure governed by what was seen by many as an outdated and harsh code of discipline was seen to be a significant contributory factor to the continuing problems with recruitment and retention. The trade union movement also became drawn into the fray. The TUC issued a Nurses Charter in 1937 which helped to publicise the long hours, poor pay and lack of long term security endured by nurses. The campaign also drew attention to the variations in terms of conditions and employment across the country and called for the establishment of nationally determined pay structures and employment rights.

The need for some kind of reform or modernisation was further amplified by the war time demand for nursing services as part of a more integrated national hospital service that could cope with the influx of both civilian and military casualties. In addition, the anticipation of increased demand for nurses after the launch of the NHS focused the attention of Government and other interested parties on the difficulties. Nursing shortages and variability in both the quantity and quality of nursing staff across the country and the way that the war drew the attention of the state towards questions relating to the nursing workforce, meant that a more sustained attempt to tackle long-standing problems would have to be made.

Making an assessment of the kind of impact that the inception of the NHS had on nursing and the success or otherwise of policy initiatives that sought to shape the profession, is quite a difficult business. The 1946 National Health Service Act and the National Health Service Act (Scotland) 1947 have often been represented as a substantial defeat for nursing. The lack of secure representation within administrative tiers of the new service and the comparatively weak position of nursing within the core health policy making community have been portrayed as evidence of the powerlessness or invisibility of nursing to policy makers and other key players. Indeed on the surface it is relatively straightforward to find evidence to support a view that nurses were subject to a form of purposeful exclusion that has distanced them from the centre of power. This can be linked to the argument that at best it is only in times of crisis caused most often by a shortage of nurses that politicians and policy makers reluctantly turn their attention to the nursing workforce.[12] While the reality is complex, I will suggest that not only have there been more chances for nurses to participate in policy change than is often recognised, but perhaps most importantly, the reasons why nurses have had such a variable and insecure relationship with the state and health politics and policy in general is not so easily explained. It is only by looking at the internal philosophies and organisation of the profession and then setting these internally driven factors against changing and essentially politically inspired demands for a certain type of nursing workforce that a true picture of the difficulties associated with nursing can be understood. This entails a recognition that nursing is a political issue in the truest sense of the term and so tied to the big questions of resource allocation and of scarcity, but is also inevitably driven by conflict and a search for compromise between competing interests. Looking at the amount of activity concerning nursing as reflected in government sponsored reports, initiatives and legislative changes over the past fifty years; it is quite hard to sustain an argument that nurses have been invisible to policy makers. Moreover, the assertion that governments only become interested in nursing because of workforce related issues of demand and supply, rather than the intrinsic and self-evident value of nursing knowledge, is in itself value laden. As the single largest and most expensive component of the NHS budget it would be a strange matter if politicians were not interested in the critical question of the existence of a safe, competent and cost effective nursing workforce that can meet the demand for nursing services across the service. In spite of this, the notion that nurses are invisible within the policy arena often forms the centrepiece of the nursing perspective. Carpenter, for example argues that for nurses invisibility underlines their subordination. While Maslin-Prothero and Masterson comment on the powerlessness on nurses in health and social care in the UK and their invisibility in key policy debates.[13]

The popularity of the invisible view of nursing has perhaps has more to do with the self- image of nursing than reality. Nurses' self-presentation has often involved an element of pathos - a view that while others threatened, bartered and accumulated, they, because of some quality integral to their calling, could do no more than patiently wait for their dedication and service to be recognised and justly rewarded. My argument is that nurses will never have the altruistic and in a sense 'pure' relationship with the state that many nurses perhaps justifiably desire. While devolution does undoubtedly open up new avenues of influence for nurses, it doesn't alter the fact that nursing leaders will still have to operate in a very challenging political environment where, now as in the past, access to core policy making communities and, perhaps more importantly, an influential position, has to be fought and bargained for and will never be freely given. This is, in one sense, a matter of nurses assuming a role which they have previously been denied or chosen to avoid. It must also be a matter of nurses developing strategies that have some chance of being attainable. In this view there is a danger that devolution and the possibility of increased fragmentation within the profession may be counter-productive to developing strategies equal to present and future challenges. As will be outlined below, nursing has in many ways flourished under a national regime, an overview which also highlights the inescapably political nature of nursing and its central importance to state policy makers. This is extremely unlikely to recede even in a more devolved system.

Nursing and the Creation of the NHS

Between 1938 and 1948 the government set up seven different committees to investigate or advise on some aspect of nursing services. This was in addition to the committee of enquiry - the Horder Committee, established by the Royal College of Nursing and the National Advisory Committee on the Nursing Profession set up by the Trades Union Congress. Some of this activity was directly related to the war effort but as the war neared its end the Ministry became more involved with looking at the specific issues relating to the provision of nursing services in the context of a National Health Service.

There was a wide range of opinion as to the cause of the nursing shortages and how best to recruit, prepare and retain sufficient numbers of nurses to meet the unknown demands of the future. The politics surrounding the issue were inevitably complicated and messy owing to the number of actors who had an interest in nursing and the range of opinion that informed their actions. In addition to the more immediate problem of shortages there were also more general questions about the implications of the NHS plans for nursing. There was no unified or coherent response from the various organisations that represented nursing interests in response to the NHS proposals. The records show that there was very little in the way of formal consultation between the Ministry of Health staff and nurse representatives; a noticeable contrast to the high level and intense negotiations which were held between the Ministry and representatives of the medical profession in the run up to the 1948 Act.[14] However, care has to be taken in interpreting why this was the case. The RCN in particular appeared to have little interest in becoming actively engaged with the Ministry of Health. They had invited Lord Horder a well known opponent of the NHS proposals to chair their own Reconstruction Committee, and there is little evidence that there was any serious attempt to develop any kind of constructive relationship with the Ministry. In fact it wasn't until 1957 when Frances Goodall who had held the post of General Secretary of the RCN since 1933 retired, that the RCN began to actively build a more stable relationship with the Ministry of Health. Until this time the RCN had, rather incongruously considering their distance from the Trade Union movement, preferred to foster relations with the Ministry of Labour.

Such insights into the politics of the day caution against offering any kind of argument that nurses were intentionally excluded from the policy making process at this time. The nursing leadership dominated as it was by matrons and ex-matrons, who may have been able to wield considerable power over their own nurses, were in the main completely inexperienced in participating in elite negotiations with government officials. If civil servants were hardly falling over themselves to incorporate nurses into the decision making process, it is also true that nurses were not knocking on the door clamouring to be admitted to the negotiating table. There was no hint that nurses could or would sabotage the new service by their opposition, as it was feared the doctors might. But more importantly, and as analysts such as Rudolf Klein have convincingly argued, it was the agreement between the state and the medical profession that became absolutely central to the whole existence of the NHS. The NHS has been, and to some extent remains, governed by a system of mutual dependency - the politics of the double bed.[15] The state was to become reliant on the doctors for the running of health policy particularly in the key area of the allocation of resources, while the doctors were to be dependent on the state not only for their income, but also for the resources at their command.[16]

The agreement between the state and the medical profession and the creation of a tight and relatively closed policy community dominated by medical interests is perhaps the single most important factor in explaining why nurses have been distanced from the centre of the policy making process. While the nursing leadership appeared ill-prepared to react to the developing situation and unwilling or unable to mount an effective challenge to the emerging NHS and articulate a clearly defined argument in support of increased nursing involvement in the policy process, it is also fair to say that state actors had no pressing reason to draw nursing into the core policy community. The state needed the co-operation of the doctors if the NHS was to get off the ground. As Smith argues: the state could act without groups, through legislative force and nationalisation but this would produce conflictual and high cost policy making.[17] Rightly or wrongly the stakes were immeasurably higher when it came to securing the agreement of the medical profession. Nursing was seen as an important and central component in the development of the new service, but interest was largely confined to the question of how to meet the demand for nurses to staff the service. Here, there was a lot of sympathy and good will shown towards nursing. Arguments in favour of improving working conditions, training and education were clearly articulated by government and other non-nursing interests. It was the nursing organisations that often appeared to have been most resistant to change. The hierarchical, some would say tyrannical, structure of nursing reflected a set of ideas and values that informed the way that influential sections of the leadership defined and projected the profession's interests. The ideals of service and associated disciplinary order which made the lives of new and junior nurses so arduous and often miserable were potent symbols of the motivations of the nursing hierarchy.[18] No women should take up the profession of nursing unless she is prepared for hard work, constant subordination of her will, and for continual self denial was the message given to new recruits as the entered one prestigious training school in 1946.[19]

In January 1946 the Ministry of Health, Department of Health for Scotland and the Ministry of Labour and National Service set up a small Working Party under the leadership of Sir Robert Wood a leading educationalist to look at the nursing needs of the new service. The Committee was also asked to consider the more fundamental question of what is the proper task of the nurse? In the end due to a disagreement between one of the Working Party members and his colleagues, a Majority and a Minority Report were produced.[20] The Reports and the subsequent reaction to their findings and recommendations stand as an informative testament of how the problems within nursing were perceived by different actors at the time. The furious debate that followed also revealed the wide range of opinion as to how nursing should be organised. Both Reports drew attention to the persistently high levels of wastage from nurse training, and focused on the internal problems within nursing. The average hospital as far as nurses were concerned was described in the Minority Report as a self-contained, segregated community of women functioning through a more or less rigid hierarchy of staff, sometimes of a quasi-military character.[21]

The long hours, poor working conditions, authoritarian atmosphere, a caste like hierarchical structure and an excessive emphasis on the performance of repetitive domestic tasks during training were all argued to contribute to recruitment difficulties and high wastage rates. A number of recommendations were made which centred on a re-orientation away from the existing apprenticeship model to a system which placed much more emphasis on education. Conditions would be made easier for student nurses and a shortened period of training would be made possible by relieving students of routine and domestic tasks. Unqualified ancillary nurses could take over many of the tasks previously performed by students. Control of the proposed new training schools was to be taken out of the hands of hospital matrons and organised on a regional basis, with training schools under a Director or Principal, and with greater input from non-nursing representatives. There were also proposals for the reform of the GNC in an attempt to make it more geographically representative, so weakening the domination of London hospital matrons, and also to strengthen representation from educational and academic interests. In essence, the Wood proposals hinted at a more flexible and modern nursing workforce, where the skills of qualified nurses would be supplemented by semi-skilled assistants whose on the job training and deployment within the workforce could be moulded to suit changing demands.[22]

The Majority Report was given a favourable reception within the Ministry of Health. In a House of Lords debate in 1948, Lord Shepherd speaking for the government said:

> Policy on the question of separation of responsibility for training from the hospitals is being considered by the Government. ... We believe that for training there should be some other authority other than merely the management of hospitals.[23]

The reaction to the Woods proposals by the nursing leadership was very mixed. Although there had long been support from some circles for the separation of training from service needs, some of the proposals elicited strident opposition. The RCN objected to the reduction in training length and the phasing out of the recently created position of assistant nurse to be replaced by an ancillary grade; and they argued in support of repetitive task performance as a successful method of learning. Both the RCN and the GNC opposed the diminished role of the hospital matron in nurse training. Unsurprisingly the GNC opposed the reduction in it's own authority which was implicit in the proposals. In their assessment of the aftermath of the Wood Report, Dingwall, Rafferty and Webster describe nursing organisations as almost Luddite in their case against proposals for educational reforms which valued the skills of the trained nurse and made a clear distinction between the qualified nurse and the unqualified helper. They suggest that nursing leaders may have been motivated in their opposition by a fear of losing control of the nursing workforce by a loosening of the strict hierarchical discipline which was seen at the time as an essential part of the experience of the trainee nurse. The rigid hierarchy, lack of personal freedom and endless repetition of seemingly futile tasks were all part of a system of discipline in which girls were purified for their calling.[24]

Significant sections of the leadership were also unwilling to support the performance of what they considered to be nursing duties by anyone other than registered nurses, assistant nurses or student nurses, and while they were willing to encourage the use of ward orderlies to perform purely domestic tasks, the prospect of the incursion of such workers into the traditional domain of the nurse aroused the strongest passions. The reality that the nursing workforce has always included a significant section of non-nurses who never the less performed some nursing tasks has been a persistent and as yet unresolved source of tension throughout the modern history of nursing.

In the end the bolder proposals concerning the restructuring of nursing were not taken forward and the opposition of the nursing organisations was an important factor in their defeat. Brian Abel-Smith in his study of the history of nursing argues that the unwillingness of the government to impose changes, which were unsupported by the nursing leadership, was indicative of the entrenched power of the profession.[25] While other factors, including the dispute between the Working Party members which weakened the impact of the main proposals must also be considered in any comprehensive explanation, it is true that the 1949 Nurses Act did not result in any major structural changes in the basic training of student nurses. The dilution of the Wood proposals in the face of opposition by nursing interests at least hints at the sensitivity of nursing policy issues for politicians. Despite the overall passivity of the nursing leadership in terms of the grand plan of the NHS, when it came to policy which more directly effected the profession, leaders were more vocal in expressing their own preferences. Policy makers were unwilling to risk alienating the nursing elite by imposing unpopular reforms. The result was that service needs continued to be the driving principle behind nurse training and innovations, which might have modernised the profession at a time of great change, were not implemented. Nursing remained inward looking, most concerned with maintaining an iron grip on the workforce through a training and professional ethos which in many respects mirrored the pattern of servitude and obedience which was first established in Florence Nightingale's time.

1950-1979: Modernisation and Modest Gains.

Especially in comparison with what was to follow, the first two decades of the NHS were marked by a certain degree of consensus. In 1958 a former

Conservative Minister of Health, was able to write that; the National Health Service, with the exception of recurring spasms about charges, is out of party politics.[26] Against this background of relative stability and optimism nursing began to develop a more confident outlook and also began a slow process of modernisation. The traditional attitude of matrons began to change; there was more support for the use of part-time nurses, male nurses and married nurses. Before the war campaigns to reduce the hours and improve the conditions of service of nurses had met with only limited success. There was a marked ambivalence amongst a section of the nursing elite to these sorts of improvements that may have challenged the vocational basis of nursing. The RCN for example had long opposed trade union attempts to regulate the hours worked by nurses. Under a nationalised system conditions did begin to improve; shorter hours, higher pay, and a superannuation scheme began to make nursing appear a less arduous occupation that demanded less in the way of personal sacrifice. Indeed nursing for thousands of women mainly from upper working class and lower middle class backgrounds for whom university education remained an unreachable prospect nursing provided an important way of securing an independent life away from home, with the promise of social advancement and a rewarding career. However, there were still shortages of nurses in some hospitals. The new nationalised regime meant that understaffed hospitals could no longer offer the inducement of a higher salary and struggled to find sufficient trained staff. Untrained staff inevitably filled the gaps left by the shortage of qualified staff particularly in the less popular hospitals for the chronic sick. By 1958 unqualified nurses falling into the category of other nursing staff amounted to a quarter of the total hospital nursing staff.[27] Clearly the grade of assistant nurse introduced after the 1943 Nurses Act had not attracted sufficient recruits to make this category of other nursing staff superfluous. A new grade of nursing auxiliary was created in 1955 amidst a debate that is very reminiscent of contemporary debates about the health care assistant. Opponents of the dilution of the nursing workforce made pleas for higher salaries for registered nurses. The 'other ranks' would then become unnecessary and once again Matrons would enjoy the pleasure of being able to choose the best applicants from an ever-increasing flow of would be nurses.[28] Supporters of the auxiliary grade took a more practical approach and recognised the need for members of staff who could relieve the pressure on trained nurses by performing basic duties.[29] However this support did not extend to a sustained commitment on behalf of the professional leadership to lobby for the provision of any kind of formal training for nursing auxiliaries. Then as now their role in the provision of nursing care was seen as something of a regrettable necessity, rather then a vital part of the total nursing service which needed to be nurtured and developed.

Nursing continued to attract the attention of policy makers in the 1960s. Partly in response to concerns about the low status of nursing and also in response to a growing awareness of problems relating to the way in which nursing services were managed, Enoch Powell, as Minister of Health, commissioned Brian Salmon to lead a small enquiry team to look into the question of the way nursing services were managed. The Salmon Committee reported in 1966 and proposed a new organisational structure that would place a nurse at every level of the NHS hierarchy as a way of improving the status and involvement of nurses in the management structure of the NHS. The new structures differentiated between top, middle and first line management. The senior nursing grades would be able to participate in the decision making process at least theoretically on a par with chief administrators and senior doctors. The lower grades were put in charge of the execution of policy at ward level. This opening out of the management structure was in part designed to reduce the autocratic power of the matrons particularly in the large acute hospitals. They were also regarded as an important indicator of professional autonomy; nurses would in future manage nurses and also have considerable freedom to develop nursing services without outside interference. At the same time, medical involvement in nurse training started to diminish and consultant doctors stopped being involved in nursing appointments. For the first time nurses had a management structure which could at least in principle give them parity with other interests in the NHS and in this respect the Salmon reforms are frequently represented as a high point in the struggle to improve the status and influence of nursing. However, even at the time, the Salmon scheme created difficulties and antagonism within nursing. The Chief Nursing Officers became distanced from the day to day running of the hospitals and the rapid introduction of the proposals meant that many nurses assuming high positions in the new structure had little in the way of management training.[30] Indeed nurse managers had a generally poor reputation by the time of the Griffiths management review in 1983. The resulting ambivalence towards nursing is thought to have contributed to the subsequent dilution of nurse representation in the new culture of general management imposed after the implementation of the Griffiths recommendations.[31]

But it was not only the organisation of nursing that attracted the attention of policy makers. At the end of the sixties nurses pay became an increasingly difficult issue for the Labour Government struggling to hold its Prices and Incomes policy together. It was against this background that Asa Briggs, a prominent historian, was asked to undertake a special investigation into nursing. The Briggs Report acknowledged that, despite rising numbers of nursing staff, all is not well with nursing. Training and education, management issues, the relationship between nursing and medicine and the public image of nursing were all seen to be problem areas. In common with previous inquiries the persistence of outdated images and ways of working was noted. Archaic styles of leadership and the negative effects of the hierarchical and autocratic structure of the profession were seen to be symptomatic of the need to move to a less formal and status conscious form of organisation.[32] Attention was also drawn to the public image of the nurse. Nursing, it was argued, retains an inherited image that belongs to the late nineteenth century.[33]

A number of recommendations were made with a view to widening the range of opportunities available to nurses that would also reflect the needs of changing NHS. The Report also called for a much clearer distinction between medicine and nursing. Where as medicine is described as diagnostic and curative the caring function of the nurse was stressed. Nursing, it was argued, should not be seen as a substitute profession for medicine but as a profession in its own right. In order to implement this agenda Briggs recommended that the various supervisory bodies responsible for pre and post registration should be disbanded, along with the General Nursing Council, and replaced with a single central regulatory body responsible for keeping the register, professional standards, education and discipline. This UK wide body would be supported by four separate national boards charged with the implementation of policies.

This key recommendation did eventually come to fruition in the 1979 Nurses, Midwifes and Health Visitors Act that created the United Kingdom Central Council (UKCC). Intense discussions and disagreements within the various factions of profession marked the lead up to the creation of the new structure. Health Visitors and Midwifes feared the domination of general nursing within a more unified organisation. Scottish nurses worried about the replacement of their largely autonomous GNC by an English dominated Central Council. Some analysts have argued that the resulting compromise contributed to the creation of a top-heavy and overly bureaucratic organisation that has perpetuated and even strengthened divisions within the profession. In fact the UKCC and four National Boards are now to be replaced by a new, smaller, UK wide council.[34]

1979 to 1998: Advance within Adversity

Looking at events since 1979 from a nursing perspective produces a confusing picture. Considering that a challenge to professional power formed a central strand of the Conservative Government's policy approach to the NHS, in some ways developments in nursing can be seen as an exception to the general trend. The establishment of the Independent Pay Review Body for nurses in July 1983 and the acceptance of the Project 2000 proposals that, after long years of campaigning, finally severed the link between training and service provision, can be seen as evidence of the advance in the professional status of nursing. Alongside this move into the higher education sector, the development of the new nursing and the associated focus on individualised and holistic patient care has fundamentally altered the way that nursing care is organised and delivered. The inclusion of the right to a named nurse as part of the Patient's Charter initiative launched by John Major's Government in 1991 was also given an enthusiastic reception by leading nurses. Lastly, the attempt to re-orient health policy towards primary care and a more inclusive definition of health encompassing preventive medicine and public health, as well as a focus on health inequalities, could also be seen as being more favourable to nursing interests as representative of a move away from the dominance of the bio-medical model of health.

However, this positive interpretation of events needs to be set against a range of other factors which point not only to the continuance of old difficulties and constraints on nursing aspirations, but also to the appearance of new challenges. The impact of managerial reforms and particularly the creation of the much maligned internal market was seen as being particularly inimical to the values and concerns of nurses.[35] Analysing the Conservative reforms from the point of view of community nurses, Walsh and Gough have argued that the contract culture of the internal market changed the status of community nursing from a loose grouping of diverse professionals with their own priorities and aspirations to a commodity.[36] Fatchett also uses the notion of nursing as a commodity in her assessment of the Conservative Government's reform program. She argues that: professional nurse practice ... has been presented as yet another manageable and marketable commodity to be promoted, **sold, brought,** discredited and even discarded in the business of NHS health care.[37] Many nurses hoped that the election of a Labour Government heralded a more favourable political climate. The recent unveiling of *Making a Difference* outlining the Government's strategic intentions for nursing, midwifery and health visiting as part of the more general modernisation of the NHS and other initiatives such as the creation of a new grade of consultant nurse, have all been greeted with enthusiasm. There is a palpable sense that there are new and important opportunities for nurses to advance their concerns in the new NHS.

However, there are questions about how far the policy climate has really changed. The assumption that the problems facing nursing under the Conservatives would ease under the new Labour government was understandable but probably over-optimistic. Analysts continue to emphasise the overall continuity in the broad thrust of Labour's health policy with the previous administration. The move from competition to planning in the NHS for example, was well under way in the final years of the Conservative Government. Other areas of change such as clinical governance also builds on previous initiatives including medical audit and the increasing drive towards evidence based medicine.[38] Chris Ham has recently argued that Labour's application of third way principles in relation to the NHS appears to be a pragmatic approach, attempting to combine the best from the market approach of the Conservatives and the hierarchical approach of old Labour.[39] Furthermore, as one fairly typical newspaper headline observed, Labour's NHS dreams turned sour remarkably quickly.[40] The constant air of crisis that pervades discussions about the NHS is perhaps the most obvious connection between the old and the new.

Conclusion

The most pressing areas of tension and concern in the present climate are ones that effect the health care system as a whole. Rationing for example, which is now never far from the headlines, is a very public and hotly debated reality that ends the myth of a fully comprehensive and national service. Furthermore, there is an acute and unresolved tension between Labour's commitment to maintaining a truly national health service, which minimises variations in the availability of services across the country, and the emphasis on diversity and local solutions to local problems at the heart of devolution. Even in those areas such as public health and the hope that under a devolved system more can be done to tackle health inequalities is fraught with difficulties. The mounting evidence that health is closely linked to social and environmental influences has led to an increasing emphasis on public health and measures specifically aimed at reducing health inequalities. But welcome and necessary though such policies are they do not in any way reduce the fundamental importance of the more formal healthcare system. In spite of this relentless expansion in the definition of health and healthcare, the general public expect curative high technology medicine to be available. Judging by the furore caused by any attempts to rationalise hospital services by closing local hospitals, there is no discernible public support for any contraction of core NHS services. For good reasons, nurses have aligned themselves with a more inclusive social model of health, but such an allegiance should not detract from involvement in debates about how nursing may need to adapt to the demands of high technology medicine and other changes in medical practice.

There are other areas where nurses may be in danger of distancing themselves from the developing political agenda in relation to health care. The demise of the internal market and the emphasis on collaborative working may have come as a welcome relief for many nurses who feel they fared badly under the Conservative years. In particular management appears to have assumed a particularly low status amongst many nurses. The ideal of the hands on nurse has been steadfastly maintained and it is the nurse that stays at the bedside who remains the symbol of the dedication and commitment of the profession. However, management appears as vital a component in the new NHS as it did in the old. In the long run nurses will suffer if management tasks continue to be seen as a regrettable necessity and are not recognised as being just as vital as direct contact with a patient.

There are other pressing problems that need to be addressed by nurses. The shortage of nurses in some areas has helped to spark off a wide-ranging debate about nursing. There are concerns about the suitability of a university based academic education for a practically based occupation. Important questions about what kind of nursing workforce is appropriate and achievable in terms of meeting the changing demands of the health care system remain as yet unanswered. In addition the slow, but unstoppable erosion of medical power and the gradual opening of the secret garden of medicine is already leading to a substantial re-evaluation of nurses' actual and potential contribution to health and health care. However, any such re-evaluation depends on taking into account the other powerful factors that are shaping change, not least the demand for a cost effective, flexible and accountable nursing workforce. In the context of devolution, although it is early days, it is hard to see these very difficult issues being tackled effectively at a local rather than a national level without introducing a potentially unstoppable process of fragmentation. In this respect it is an interesting observation that nurses in Australia who work within a federal system of government where each state and territory has its own Nursing Act and hence significant local differences from one state to another, report that they work hard to offset any tendency towards fragmentation by having strong national organisations to represent nursing interests and present a unified response to national issues.

Nursing will remain a crucial element in any of the future post devolution health care system. Whether or not significant differences evolve between health services in different part of the UK is, in the context of the argument presented here, of less importance for the long term development of nursing than finding new ways of engagement with the wider forces shaping change in our health care system. Consideration of the development of nursing since the start of the NHS reveals how it is inevitably and intimately connected to the changing and intensely political nature of the health care system as a whole.

There is no convenient dividing line between the professional and the political in the NHS. Nurses need to develop a more pragmatic understanding of the constraints as well as the opportunities that face them. Devolution will no doubt present nurses with new opportunities to influence and shape change, however there is nothing fixed. Professional definitions of merit are now even more than in the past likely to be challenged, and can not be relied upon as a guarantee of consultation in the decision making process. Nurses will have to maximise their political skills in order to meet the challenges that lie ahead. Unity not fragmentation provides the most promising option in the turbulent times ahead.

Notes

1   Dingwall, Rafferty and Webster, *An Introduction to the Social History Of Nursing*, London, Routledge, (1991).

2   See for example Leys, C. 'The NHS after Devolution', *British Medical Journal*, 318: 1155-56, (1999).

3   'Nurse Leadership in Scotland an interview with June Andrews', *Nursing Management* Vol. 6 No 7, (November 1999).
4   Scottish Office Press Release, (26 Nov 1999).
5   A review of the contribution of nurses to improving the public's health was started in 1999 and aims to report in autumn 2000. See Health Bulletin from the Chief Nursing Officer, Scottish Executive, (January 2000).
6   Francis, B. and Humphreys J, *Devolution or Centralization in Nurse Education Today*, 18, (1998), pp.433-439.
7   Hazell R, and Jervis P. *Devolution and Health*, London, Nuffield Trust, (1998).
8   Hazell R, and Jervis P. *Devolution and Health*, London, Nuffield Trust, (1998), p.324.
9   The European Oncology Nursing Society (EONS) provides a good example of a highly effective European nursing organization. See: *Report of the Masterclass on Nursing and Europe*, The Scottish Office, Department of Health, (1998).
10   See for example Davies, C. *Gender and the Professional Predicament in Nursing*, Buckingham, Open University Press. An influential account of gender in relation to nursing power and influence, (1995).
11   The report of the Athlone Committee set up by the Ministry of Health in 1937 found that many of the recruits into nursing came from lower middle and upper working class backgrounds and needed to work if they were not to marry. This contrasted with the aspirations of the nursing elite to attract girls from solidly middle class families who would be less motivated by financial concerns. See also Wise, A.R.J. *Your Hospital*, London, Willman Heinemann, (1949).
12   See Rafferty, A. M. 'Nursing Policy and the nationalization of nursing: the representation of 'crisis' and the 'crisis' of representation', in Robinson, J, Gray, A, and Elkan, R. *Policy Issues in Nursing*, Milton Keynes: Open University Press, (1992).
13   Carpenter, M. *The subordination of nurses in health care in Riska and Wegar, Gender Work and Medicine*, London Sage, (1993). Maslin-Prothero, S. and Masterson, A. 'Continuing Care: Developing a Policy Analysis for Nursing', *Journal of Advanced Nursing*, vol. 28, no 3, (1998), pp.548-553.
14   See Scott E.J.C. *The Influence of the Staff of the Ministry of Health on policies for nursing 1919-1968* (1994) for a very comprehensive review of the role and influence of the Ministry of Health on the development of nursing policies.
15   Klein, R. 'The State and the Profession: the politics of the double bed', *British Medical Journal*, 301, 3:700-702, (1990).
16   Klein R. 'The State and the Profession: the politics of the double bed', *British Medical Journal*, 301, 3:700-702, (1990).
17   Smith, M. *Pressure Power and Policy*, Harvester Wheatsheaf, (1993).
18   John Cohen's Minority Report on the Recruitment and Training of Nurses published in 1948 continues a number of articulate and graphic accounts of the hardships and of the harsh discipline and isolation from the outside world that had to be endured by nurses at this time.
19   Rivett G *From Cradle to grave Fifty Years of the NHS*, London, Kings Fund, (1998).
20   The Minority Report was written by Dr John Cohen a psychologist who had worked in the Cabinet Office. He objected to a lack of scientific method in the

approach of his colleagues. Cohen urged a more systematic and scientific approach to policy-making and argued that nursing problems could only be solved if placed in the context of wider health service developments. Ministry of Health Department of Health For Scotland and Ministry of Labor and National Service, *Working Party on the Recruitment and Training of Nurses. Minority Report*, (1948).

21   Ministry of Health Department of Health For Scotland and Ministry of Labor and National Service, *Working Party on the Recruitment and Training of Nurses. Minority Report*, (1948), p47.

22   See Dingwall, Rafferty and Webster *An Introduction to the Social History of Nursing*, (1991).

23   Abel Smith, B. *A History of the Nursing Profession*, London, Heinemann, (1960), p.216.

24   Dingwall, Rafferty and Webster *An Introduction to the Social History of Nursing*, (1991), p.118.

25   Abel Smith, B. *A History of the Nursing Profession*, London, Heinemann, (1960), p.227.

26   Klein, R. The New Politics of the NHS, (1995), p.29.

27   Abel Smith, B. *A History of the Nursing Profession*, London, Heinemann, (1960), p.235.

28   Taken from the British Journal of Nursing, July 1955 quoted in Abel Smith, B *A History of the Nursing Profession*, London, Heinemann, (1960), p.236.

29   Nursing Times 17 June 1955, in Abel Smith, B. *A History of the Nursing Profession*, London, Heinemann, (1960), p.236.

30   Rivett, G. *From Cradle to grave Fifty Years of the NHS*, London, Kings Fund, (1998), p.261.

31   Strong, P. and Robinson, J. *The NHS Under New Management*, Buckingham, Open University Press, (1990).

32   Asa Briggs (chairman), Report of the committee on nursing, London, HMSO, (1971).

33   Asa Briggs (chairman), Report of the committee on nursing, London, HMSO, (1971), pp.23-24.

34   See the J.M Consulting Ltd., *Report on a review of the Nurses, Midwives and Health Visitors Act*, 1998 and Department of Health, *Review of the Nurses, Midwives and Health Visitors Act: Government Response to the recommendations*, London, HMSO, (1999).

35   Fatchett, A. *Politics, Policy and Nursing*, London, Balliere Tindall, (1994).

36   Walsh,N. and Gough,P. 'From Profession to Commodity', *Nursing Times*, 93, 30, (1997), pp.37-43.

37   Fatchet,A. *Nursing in the New NHS: Modern Dependable*, London, Balliere Tindall, (1998), p. 153.

38   Klein, R. 'Why Britain is re-organising its National Health Service - yet again', *Health Affairs* 17, 4, (1998), pp.111-125.

39   Ham, C. 'The third way in health' *Journal of Health Service Research and Policy*, 4, 3, (1999), pp.168-173.

40   *The Guardian*, 10 Sept 1997.

5. Fifty Years in the Battle for Public Health. An interview with Dr. David Player

DAVID PLAYER WITH CHRIS NOTTINGHAM

It would be difficult to imagine anyone with a more extensive and varied experience of the National Health Service than David Player. Although he is perhaps best known as a public health campaigner, his professional experience stretches from dermatology to psychiatry, encompassing general practice, infectious diseases, obstetrics, and much else along the way. He was educated at Calder Street School and Bellahouston Academy and then went to study medicine at Glasgow University, graduating in 1949. He gained greatest prominence as Director of the Scottish Health Education Group between 1973 and1982 and as Director General of the Health Education Council from 1982 until 1987 when that body, in the midst of fierce public controversy, was closed down by Margaret Thatcher's Government. One of his final acts in the latter position was to host one of the most unusual press conferences ever held to launch the report, *The Health Divide*, which he had commissioned from Margaret Whitehead. An hour before the conference was due to take place the chair of the HEC had decided that the report was too controversial and forbade David from attending. Nothing daunted he set off with both panel and journalists and the launch eventually took place in a room behind a guitar shop in Soho, lent by the Disability Alliance. Since his retirement as District Medical Officer of the South Birmingham Health Authority in 1991 David has remained a tireless combatant for the values of public health and has at the same time managed to successfully complete an honours degree in history at St. Andrews University. He only recently retired as Chair of the Public Health Alliance and is still Honorary Visiting Professor in the Department of Clinical Epidemiology and General Practice at the Royal Free Hospital School of Medicine. He remains, as participants in the NHS 50 Conference will testify, a combative and engaging campaigner for the cause.

What first convinced you that public health approach was the right one?

It was personal experience more than anything else. My background had always disposed me towards a social understanding of medicine and health. I always saw politics and medicine as inevitably intertwined but it was my experience as general practitioner in West Cumberland in the late 1950s, which focussed my interests. My commitment to prevention arose from experience in my first stint as a GP.

Cumberland will evoke images of lakes and mountains but the communities in which I worked could not have been more different; they were the back kitchen of the Lake District; communities which were based on coal and ironstone mining. The villages were very different in some respects. The population of Cleator Moor, for instance, was of Irish Catholic origin while that of Egremont was mainly Anglican. Some worked in the coal mines, others with the ironstone, but while different in these respects they were united in the grim legacy of bad health associated with these occupations. In those days also there was no compensation for diseases such as pneumoconiosis and haemosiderosis, which were widespread. I was prescribing oxygen for many of my patients simply so that they could get to the toilet. It was easy enough to see that the work of a doctor in such circumstances was only patching up. The only cure would be to change the conditions that were obviously producing the illness in the first place.

I remember clearly when I decided that I could no longer go along with it. It was a miserable winter Saturday. I was called out to a patient in Frizington, a wretched one street mining town. This patient, like so many others, was a middle-aged man debilitated with chronic chest disease, which had flared up into acute bronchitis. As usual I prescribed more oxygen, more antibiotic and arranged to call back in the morning. As I looked round the room I noticed that his wife had arranged pots and pans across the floor to catch the rain which was dripping through the ceiling. I suddenly thought, "What am I doing here? What this man needs is decent house and a different job." I decided there and then go back to Glasgow to do the diploma in public health.

How did that work then?

There were about 20 in class, all of them doctors. Professor Ferguson, who was quite famous, was our teacher. The course involved classes, tutorials and visits and was full time, nine to five. One of the conditions for being accepted onto the course was that we must not take on any work, we all had to agree to that. But that was no use to me. I was a married man and needed the money. I took a job at a Paisley Fever and Chest Hospital being on call from six in the evening until eight the next morning. I took admissions, did ward rounds and wrote up case notes. I also took on locum work for GP's in the area. Sometimes I signed people into hospital as a locum GP and admitted them to hospital later that same day. Nonetheless I was the gold medal student. I wrote my thesis on suicide, applying Durkheim's ideas from 'Le Suicide'.

After this the logical step was to a job as Medical Officer of Health?

I went to Dumfries. The process of appointment of the Medical Officer in those days was rather awesome. The Provost accompanied by some twenty councillors appointed me. I had an early lesson in the independence of the MOH in the Scottish system. The Provost was a butcher and I discovered that the Sanitary Inspector had lodged an unfavourable report after an inspection of his shop, so the day after he had appointed me my first task was to shut him down. He didn't like it but just had to put up with it. While the Council appointed the MOH he could only be dismissed by the Secretary of State for Scotland.

During my time in Dumfries we introduced some of the most progressive things in Britain such as screening for cervical and breast cancer. Our Consultant Pathologist Dr. Nancy Scott had worked with Dr. Papanicolou who had developed smear testing in the United States. We screened all the women in Dumfries and our gynaecologist, Dr. Bruce Dewar, operated. We were the first to do this.

We were also the first in Scotland to have all health visitors, midwives and physiotherapists attached to general practice; first also to have a purpose built centre to cater for the mental and physically handicapped. However, our attempts to build a purpose built health centre ran into trouble from medical conservatism. The opposition of the GP's was based on the fact that they associated such things with Local Authorities. One GP, perhaps associating the idea with luncheon clubs complained that he was not going to have the "smell of soup" interfering with his diagnosis. The doctors however were mostly motivated by the horror of being under Local Authority councillors.

Your next move was to the Scottish Office

I was keen to work with Sir John Brotherton who was Chief Medical Officer at the Scottish Home and Health Department. He was a giant of the public health movement. The trailblazing in Dumfries had attracted attention and, as I also had psychiatric qualifications, I applied when a job came up to develop a programme for mental health for Scotland. As it turned out I was the only applicant.

Unfortunately the day I started, Sir John was on holiday and his deputy was in charge. Instead of developing the mental health programme I became medical and psychiatric advisor to the Secretary of State on the Prison and Borstal service. I did this for three and a half years and it was a most depressing job.

How did the move to the Health Education Unit come about?

Smoking was killing more people than any other preventable disease and Sir John was determined to do something about it. The Director of the Health Education Unit had gone to London and I was offered the job. I was initially in two minds about taking it as health education had a rather soft image but I was tempted by the fact that I would be my own boss and have a free hand and a large budget. It was after all, an opportunity to raise the importance of health.

Initially it was decided to target male smokers. This was possibly a mistake but male rates of smoking were then three or four times higher than female. I began thinking about how to get at the problem. What was important to men? I thought of sport and particularly of football. The next idea came about by chance. I was on a train from Dumfries to Glasgow and fell into conversation with some guys who were playing cards and drinking. It turned out that one of them was the scout for St. Mirren who were at that time managed by Alex Ferguson. We talked about Bill Shankly the manager of Liverpool who had recently been interviewed on TV. He'd said he wouldn't have a smoker in his team because his figures showed that so many games were decided in the last ten minutes and the ability of players to go at the same speed throughout the game depended on them being totally fit and not smoking.

I went to see Ferguson and offered to sponsor them if they would become a non-smoking team. When they were playing the last game of the season for the championship we put up thousands for them to wear kit saying they were a non-smoking team. We had photographs prepared with the slogan 'champions don't smoke'. This hit the headlines. When Ferguson went to Aberdeen we did the same deal with them. We got everyone involved from the Minister of Health to Miss Scotland.

You also became involved with the national team?

We got our best publicity through sponsoring Scotland as the No Smoking Team in the World Cup in Spain in 1982. I first went to see Ernie Walker who was Secretary of the SFA. I'd been at the same school as him and he had the reputation of being a real hard man. His basic question was always how much money was in it for them. We initially allocated £75,000 to the SFA and the players but the final bill was around £400,000.

Jock Stein the manager was a true believer and always co-operated. Once in Spain we got other teams to sign up. We got help from the Brazilians, the Russains and the Czechs. We built a huge hot air balloon with the Scottish lion and the no smoking logo on the sides and flew it above the grounds every time Scotland played. We also targeted the Scottish fans. Some of them did still smoke but they were very apologetic about it. This was the season when the Scottish fans became 'the angels' because of their good behaviour compared with the other fans - especially the English.

Jock Stein was a total supporter. We went round some of the biggest schools in Scotland to address assemblies. Jock was the best propagandist we could imagine. He once said to a large assembly in a secondary school in Lanarkshire that it would give him more pleasure if Scottish youngsters stopped smoking than if Scotland won the world cup. We took him along to Radio Clyde to say it on tape for a 15 second commercial. He never accepted money for it.

You were also keen on getting health education into the universities?

We helped to fund lectureships and chairs in most of the Scottish universities. For example we funded a lectureship in psychology at Strathclyde University which eventually formed the Department of Media

Studies. They viewed and tested leaflets and TV commercials. This was essentially pump priming to establish health education as a profession.

How successful do you feel the anti-smoking campaign was?

Smoking rates certainly did begin to come down but it's difficult to deal in terms of cause and effect because of the many associated factors. It did though, give me a very clear insight into the activities of what I call the enemies of health or enemies of the people; in particular the tobacco and drink industries. Our activities were always going to affect their interests, such as when Scotland took the lead in banning alcohol from football grounds. The tobacco and drinks industries did not like it. I was once called the Ayatollah Khomeni of Scotland by some members of the Scotch Whisky Association. When we took over sponsorship of the Scottish League Cup we banned all alcohol adverts in grounds and in programmes.

There never seemed any point in meeting the tobacco people but I was always prepared to look for common ground with the alcohol industry. Our aim in Scotland was to reduce both per capita as well as total consumption. The degree of harm goes up as the per capita consumption goes up. Our meetings always broke down because their aim was always to increase consumption. They were prepared to support sensible drinking but they didn't want this to result in a reduction of sales. This was the crunch.

When I had my going away party at the Royal College of Physicians in Edinburgh one of the alcohol industry men was there. He told me jokingly, "I've come along to make sure you're leaving the damned country."

The pressure must have been even greater when you went to the Health Education Council in London?

The tobacco industry alone had about forty MPs who would get up and rubbish any report that came out on the dangers of smoking. They had good friends in government as well. In 1994 they put up £11.5 million for health research. Money was offered to universities up and down the country through the Health Promotion Research Trust set up with this cash from the tobacco industry. The research thus funded had a condition that it must not look at the effects of tobacco. Very distinguished professors and departments of public health applied. Very few were immune. We warned that those who took the money could expect no more money from us. Such vested interests are very powerful and they can intervene at any level. I wonder how far it is a coincidence that Kenneth Clark once a Minister of Health is now Deputy Chairman of British American Tobacco and that Mrs. Thatcher's Foundation gets a lot of its funds from tobacco companies. The first scandal to hit the Blair government was when they gave way to Bernie Ecclestone and continued to allow cigarette advertising on Formula 1 racing cars.

How did your dismissal come about?

In 1986, when speaking at a conference at Green College in Oxford I got a phone call from my number two telling me that something was happening and I'd better get back to London as soon as possible. I was told that officials from the Department of health would visit me at ten the next morning. I hadn't a clue what it was about and our Chairman wouldn't say. We all met the next morning and were chatting away quite pleasantly though they didn't give any clue as to why they were there. Then at exactly 10 o'clock one of them took a sheet out of brief case and said this is what Secretary of State, Norman Fowler, would be reading out at the same time in Parliament. It was the announcement that the Health Education Council was being wound up and replaced by a new organisation, the Health Education Authority which was constituted as a special Health Authority. Because of AIDS the government realised that it was going to have to put a lot more money into health education and the HEC was a quango. They felt they needed an organisation that they could control more directly. Everyone in the HEC had to reapply for jobs with the new organisation. All were offered re employment, apart from myself. I applied for the post as new Director General but was not entirely surprised when I was unsuccessful. It was clear that my opposition to the Tobacco, Alcohol and Food industries had made me very unpopular. They knew I was basically anti-capitalist, but they had trouble getting rid of me. They couldn't do the expenses trick, which is what they often used, and I refused offers of Fellowships and similar bribes so they had to take this opportunity. It became something of a *cause celebre*.

The Blair Government has made a lot of positive noises about public health. Aren't there causes for optimism?

On the face of it there seemed to be reason for hope. The Chancellor is on record in his book *Scotland: the Real Divide*, which he edited with Robin Cook, as believing that redistribution of wealth is fundamental and that nothing worthwhile can be achieved in the fight against poverty and inequalities in health without substantial moves in that direction.

Tessa Jowell became the first minister for public health but she was far less receptive to the idea of the need for redistributive taxes. We did meet with her but she recommended that we had to be 'realistic' and beware of creating a dependency culture.

The New Labour record though, can only be described as terrible. To defend financial constraints is not good enough. At the end of the last war in 1945 the country was bankrupt but we managed to introduce the welfare state. The difference between then and now is that the political will was there in the aftermath of the war. Free milk for school children was actually brought in during the Second World War. We even managed to stand up to the drink industry and regulate sales during the First World War. In 1945 there was very little money but massive political will. So much of what is now being done, such as decreasing taxes on businessmen's share options, is actually promoting inequality. This happens at the same time as we are decreasing benefits to single mothers. This was a very important incident and Malcolm Chisholm M.P. deserves great credit for resigning his ministerial post over it. That was a very brave gesture. There are now even attempts to cut benefits for the disabled.

We've had the Acheson Report. At least we can now talk about inequalities and health but there is no discussion of the large-scale redistribution that is needed to make an impact. The rhetoric of social exclusion is fine but among the first things the Social Exclusion Unit came up with was giving the police the power to apprehend truants in the street and fining families for bad behaviour. We've recently had Louise Casey, the tsarina of rough sleepers, complaining that giving people good sleeping bags and feeding them is really doing them a disservice and just encouraging them to sleep rough. It's also significant that when Yvette Cooper replaced Tessa Jowell as public health minister the post was downgraded. It does seem that public health is being put on the back burner and demoted.

One of New Labour's greatest errors is to continue with the Private Finance Initiative, now renamed the Public Private Partnership. This is getting into bed with big business; the selling of a birthright; short termism of the worst kind. It may look good at first sight but some of the contracts run for the next thirty years. The Health Service will be paying at an extortionate rate throughout the next generation. Yet New Labour seems deeply wedded to it. When Frank Dobson was challenged over it he dismissed all criticism and said it was "the only show in town". Alan Milburn is no less committed. At a recent meeting at the Royal College of Physicians he, unusually, agreed to answer questions off the cuff. When challenged on the effects of the Public Private Partnership by a well-respected researcher he seemed to lose the place and, in front of a distinguished audience told his questioner it was time he grew up. New Labour in many respects seems just as hostile to the public service as their predecessors. In this they are missing a real opportunity.

Does the coming of the Scottish Parliament represent an opportunity to advance the public health agenda this side of the border?

Scotland is more socialist and New Labour is less entrenched here. There are some signs of willingness to resist what is going on in Westminster. The Parliament does make it more difficult to overrule Scottish opinion. However if there is an opportunity it must be taken now. There is potential for action but there may not be in a year's time. It will require boldness and they will need to take on London. Student fees might prove to be the precedent. If they do this there is the possibility of a new alignment in Scotland which will support a radical approach to the redistribution of wealth. In public health terms this is now the key issue. The anti smoking campaign was always going to take on its own momentum once smokers became a minority of the population and passive smoking was accepted as an issue. All our efforts must now be devoted to inequalities of health and poverty. That's the big one.

6. Whatever Happened to the *Occupational* Health Service? The NHS, the OHS and the asbestos tragedy on Clydeside

RONALD JOHNSTON AND ARTHUR McIVOR

Since its inception in 1948 the NHS has been synonymous with the welfare state. Harold Wilson called it 'the very temple of our social security system', and for Michael Foot it was 'the greatest Socialist achievement of the Labour government.'[1] The main debate regarding the NHS has centred around the degree of health care inequalities which it failed to eradicate, and the notion that the middle classes have historically derived more benefit from state health provision is a strong and compelling one.[2] A forgotten factor of this debate, though, is that one of the main reasons for the relative poor health of the working class is that it has had to endure more dangerous and unhealthy working conditions than any other class. This chapter will illustrate how this causal factor has never been adequately addressed by state welfarism, and that this neglect is reflected in the state's failure to establish an occupational health service (OHS) within the National Health Service (NHS) - thus meeting work-determined health inequalities head on. It will be argued that the NHS's emphasis on cure rather than prevention resulted in the work wounded being patched up and returned to unsafe working environments, and that little positive contribution was made to addressing the root causes of occupation-related disease, mortality and morbidity from work-related disease. Using the currently unfolding asbestos tragedy on Clydeside as an exemplar, it will be argued here that the rate of disability and mortality could have been drastically reduced if occupational medicine had been given a greater priority within the post-1945 Welfare State.

The development of occupational health services

Concern over occupational health has a long history. Hippocrates in 355 BC commented upon the dangers of working with lead. Later, Pliny mentions how those working with vermilion covered their faces with a loose bladder as a precaution against inhalation of harmful dust. However, the first serious study of occupational health was conducted by the Italian physician Ramazinni in 1700. Ramazinni dedicated 40 years of research into classifying 100 occupationally caused diseases, stressed the need for the physician to know the occupation of the patient, and recommended that occupational health should be established as a separate discipline.[3]

In Britain, the evolution of occupational health has lagged well behind the development of industrial capitalism. In the eighteenth century some pioneering physicians took an interest in the health risks connected to certain work processes - such as the tendency for chimney sweeps to contract scrotal cancer, and for bakers to succumb to skin disease. With industrialisation and urbanisation in the 19th century, influential individuals such as Robert Owen, Sir Robert Peel, and the Earl of Shaftsbury, campaigned for measures to protect workers' health. The Factory Act of 1803 gave JPs the power to appoint factory visitors. The first appointed government factory inspectors came on the scene in 1833; and were given wider powers in 1855. However, it was not until the end of the nineteenth century - well after the pinnacle of British industrial prominence had been reached - that the first Medical Inspector of Factories was appointed and legislation allowed 'Certifying Surgeons' to investigate cases of industrial disease and to undertake regular medical examinations of workers deemed especially at risk. These changes were amongst a cluster of reforms emerging from the Dangerous Trades Committees of the 1890s. The 1897 Workmen's Compensation Act - which held employers liable for the safety of their staff - also provided further impetus to a general improvement in industrial welfare.

The pattern throughout the 19th century, then, was one of slow and limited state intervention in occupational health - and recent work has also highlighted the error of assuming an upward curve of improvement in relation to industrial compensation.[4] Despite awareness that most work had some sort of unhealthy side effect, the evolution of British laissez faire capitalism ensured that the pursuit of profit generally took precedence over any attempts to cultivate a healthier working environment.[5] The first serious attempt to compensate workers for industrial diseases - the amended Workmen's Compensation Act of 1906 - covered only six prescribed diseases where the link between work and disability or death was irrefutable. Before the First World War, then, disability caused by the most significant of occupational hazards -the inhalation of harmful dust - was neither prescribed nor compensatable. Inevitably this caused wide variations in life chances relating to occupation, as table 1 below illustrates.

Table 1

Comparative mortality of selected male workers, 1880-2

	All causes	Lung & respiratory Disease
Agriculture, fishing, clergy	100	100
Grocers	139	130
Coal miners	160	148
Masons, builders, bricklayers	174	208
Wool workers	186	203
Tailors	189	217
Cotton workers	196	250
Quarrymen	202	268
Cutlers	235	350
File makers	300	360
Earthenware workers	313	514
Cornish metal miners	331	528

Source: Evidence of Dr W. Ogle, *Royal Commission on Labour, Digest of Evidence*, June 1893, C7063, 1893, pp. 38-40.

The interface between medical knowledge and occupational health has also been slow to form. It was not until the First World War that industrial medicine was taught in British universities; the first occupational health journal only appeared in the early 1940s - at which time the first post graduate qualification on occupational health was offered to doctors.[6] Moreover, despite the fact the 1944 White Paper on the NHS spoke of a need for 'proper postgraduate training of GP's who are going to engage in industrial or other specialities', nothing much was done along these lines.[7] Indeed four years after the creation of the NHS the average time devoted to

occupational health at medical schools within the whole degree course was
6 - 8 lectures - and these were normally part of a series of lectures on public
health and social medicine.[8]

The two wars stimulated awareness of the importance of a healthy
workforce, but the main driving force was the need for increased
productivity. A 1951 government report made this clear: 'It was then
[during the First World War] that it was fully realised that the health of the
worker is a factor of great economic value and that if he were to achieve
maximum efficiency as a producer he must be maintained in good health.'[9]
During the first war many factories came under the control of the Ministry
of Munitions - which had its own medical department to advise on
industrial hygiene - and important studies were carried out by the Health of
Munitions Workers' Committee and, after 1917, the Industrial Health
Research Board, on the effect of work on health.

In the inter-war period the connection between good health and
higher productivity was further examined, and this was accompanied by
greater emphasis on industrial safety.[10] Some employers began appointing
doctors as whole or part-time industrial medical officers, and the 1937
Factories Act stipulated that workshops and factories should have first aid
equipment on the premises in the care of a responsible person - who, in
premises that employed more than 50 people, had to be trained in first aid.
This act also gave the Secretary of State the power to insist that companies
establish OHS's - a form of state intervention that was never exercised.[11]
During the Second World War there was an even greater interest in the
medical supervision of the workforce. Once again, though, this stemmed
from a need to ensure maximum war production, and not from a desire to
protect workers from dangerous processes. As in the First World War many
factories came under government control, and it was in these premises that
concern over workers' health was most strongly developed. In 1940 the
Factories (Medical and Welfare Services) Order gave the Chief Inspector of
Factories the power to order - where he or she thought necessary - factory
owners to employ a factory doctor, or nurse; while in the private sphere,
many employers also expanded their medical services.[12] As a result of the
1940 Order a large number of doctors with no training in occupational
health became involved with industry. Turnover was heavy, however, and
few of these 'war doctors' remained in their posts after the war.[13]

Despite the impetus provided by the two world wars, then,
occupational health in Britain was still poorly developed by 1948. A body
of legislation had been passed aimed at protecting groups of workers from

risk: such as the Factory Acts and Mines Acts; the Explosives Acts of 1915 and 1923; the Wool, Goat Hair and Camel Hair Regulations of 1907; the Bakehouses Welfare Order of 1927; and the Petroleum (Consolidation) Act of 1928. But their coverage of the British workforce was patchy - for example, agriculture was not covered by any health and safety laws until 1956.

The Medical Factory Inspectorate comprised 15 inspectors and came under the auspices of the Ministry of Labour and National Service. Part of the Inspectorate's mandate was to investigate cases of industrial disease and examine dangerous work processes. However, it was also expected to keep pace with scientific knowledge regarding occupational health, and liase with other government departments - among them the Department of Health for Scotland. These obligations - and the fact that there were only 15 inspectors - meant the bulk of occupational health work was carried out by the next stratum of the service: the Appointed Factory Doctors (AFDs). These were a continuation of the Certifying Surgeons initiated in the Victorian period, and in the early 1940s, 1800 of them were responsible for the workplace health of the entire nation - assisted by 175 whole-time occupational health doctors, and around 700 other doctors who dealt with occupational health on a part-time basis only.[14] Each of the AFD's served a particular district, and most of them also ran their own general practices within the NHS after 1948. The shortcomings of the system were noted in 1949 when it was estimated that 1400 of the 1800 AFD's only worked 3 hours a week in a factory.[15] Moreover, due to their background and education they tended to share the same values as the factory management. One AFD writing of the importance of industrial medicine in a GP's journal made this clear when he referred to the factory doctor as 'one of the highest grades in the works' hierarchy.' Consequently, he argued that medical inspections should be thorough and meticulous, as 'this is the first time that the new starter will see one of the firm's high officials at work.'[16] As well as the AFD's there were also around 2500 State Registered Nurses and 1400 other nursing staff employed in factories throughout Britain. This was a very small number compared to those employed in general health services - there were 27,500 nurses employed in Scotland alone in 1951.

The coming of the NHS

The initiation of the NHS in 1948 meant Britain once again led the world by providing free medical care to its entire population. This exclusivity was retained until the establishment of Sweden's National Health Service two decades years later. With the coming of the NHS the 'partial and muddled patchwork' of British health care was replaced by a coherent manageable system.[17] However, Bevan deliberately omitted coverage of industrial health in his plans - according to one commentator, this was because he was aware that his project was already ambitious enough.[18] Jones has argued that disagreement among the key players in the planning stage resulted in the creation of what was in effect a national hospital service, largely out of touch with the changing health needs of the nation. For Jones, though, the biggest failure was the omission in 1948 of an OHS built into the NHS structure.[19] This omission meant the historic separation of work from health was now institutionalised, that the scope of British occupational health remained fragmentary, and that its future development would be stilted.

In the years leading up to the initiation of the NHS there had been growing evidence that an OHS was urgently required. In 1945 the Royal College of Physicians (RCP) had drawn attention to the fact that most people spent around a third of their lives at work; recommended that a holistic approach to health was needed; and that this necessitated the establishment of an OHS.[20] Long after the initiation of the NHS the RCP and the Medical Commission on Accident Prevention continued to argue for the establishment of an OHS within the NHS.[21] In 1941 the British Medical Association's (BMA) report 'Industrial Health in Factories' had advocated a closer link between medicine and industry. Twenty years later the BMA was still making the same appeal. A Privy Council Committee in 1947 highlighted the failures of pre-war voluntarism in occupational health, criticising British employers for not taking up the progressive message from the 'human factor' theorists and hence jeopardising the war effort.[22] In 1949 the Dale Committee examined the potential overlap between occupational health provision and that offered by the NHS. Its principal findings were that the OHS was complementary to that provided by the NHS, but that both systems should be co-ordinated.[23] This was also the recommendation of the Gowers Committee, which sat at the same time. It looked, then, as though an OHS was on the way, and a writer in the

Glasgow Herald warmly welcomed the imminent setting up of the new service in 1951.[24]

Organised labour also called upon the government to pay more attention to occupational health. It has been argued that where occupational health and safety was concerned, British trade unions have historically prioritised other issues - such as wages and hours.[25] This could well be an over-generalisation as recent research has shown that this charge cannot really be levelled at the TUC and the STUC in respect to occupational health by the 1940s.[26] In 1944 the TUC held discussions with the Royal College of Physicians over proposals to introduce lectures on occupational health to medical undergraduates and postgraduates. A year later, during the planning stage of the NHS, the TUC strongly urged that a comprehensive OHS be established 'complementary to and integrated within the NHS.' Shortly after the war the government promised the TUC that once a large enough cadre of suitably qualified doctors was built up an industrial medical service would be established.[27]

The General Council of the TUC fully endorsed the recommendations of the Dale Committee and sent a memorandum to the Minister of Labour asking that an OHS be set up along the lines recommended by Dale. The TUC wanted a health service that would include, among other things, 'the recognition, evaluation and control of occupational hazards ... Early diagnosis of the effects of exposure to hazards ... [and] the prescription, diagnosis and assessment of occupational disease.'[28] In Scotland, the STUC fully supported the call for better health care at work. However, as late as 1972 the STUC was still urging the government to establish a comprehensive occupational health service within the NHS.[29]

Fuel was added to the fire with the growing evidence that industrial medical provision was skewed towards larger premises. A survey conducted by the Factory Inspectorate in 1958 found that only in some factories with more than 1000 workers were full-time doctors employed.[30] The Society of Occupational Medicine (SOM) represented over 1000 doctors in 1970. When the SOM gave evidence to the Robens Committee in 1972, its testimony drew attention to the lack of coverage of existing occupational health provision, and advocated that occupational health should be brought under the control of the DHSS.[31]

However, whilst governments accepted in principle these recommendations from the highest echelons of trade unionism, no further progress was made. Further, although the government agreed with the

International Labour Conference's recommendation in 1959 that a proper OHS be established, a White Paper later made clear that it would not be possible to have this in a country which already had an NHS - the following year a government publication called *Health at Work* was distributed to factory occupiers throughout Britain in an effort to encourage them to establish their *own* OHS.[32] In 1968 the Royal Commission on Medical Education stated that there would be no changes made to the provision of British occupational health.[33] And, shortly after, the Senior Medical Inspector made the government's position crystal clear: 'In British law,' he said, 'the factory occupier ... is responsible for the safety, health, and welfare of his employees, and any action he takes ... to meet these obligations is for him to decide.'[34]

A major change to occupational health and safety occurred with the passage of the Health and Safety at Work Act in 1974. However, once again an opportunity was missed. In 1972 the Robens Committee published its recommendations. This committee had been commissioned two years earlier specifically to investigate health and safety at work. Despite the weight of evidence arguing for the setting up of an OHS within the NHS, the committee concluded that such provision would only duplicate that already provided by the NHS, and recommended that the government play no further part in OHS provision. The only immediate change to the system was the setting up of the Employment Medical Advisory Service (EMAS) - which brought the network of Appointed Factory Doctors into an organisation with a wider advisory role. The Government, though, fully realised the shortfalls of EMAS scope, and the Parliamentary Under-Secretary of State stated in 1973 that

> 'the new service will not be, and is not intended to be, a comprehensive occupational health service... We already have an NHS which provides comprehensive medical care for the whole population and it would be wasteful of medical skills for the Government to duplicate this by providing general medical care in industry.'

Further, the Secretary of State for Scotland took the same view: 'Re-organisation of the NHS would be considerably complicated by the simultaneous incorporation of wide new responsibilities.'[35] As far as a national system was concerned, though, the main conclusion was that any future improvements to workplace health and safety should be the responsibility of employers and workers. It was on this recommendation that the 1974 Health and Safety at Work Act (HSWA) was based. Before turning to this legislation, though, we shall briefly illustrate how Scotland was the testing ground for a much more interventionist approach to occupational health.

Alternative approaches to intervention

The heavy concentration of industry in the Clydeside area made it an ideal location for monitoring the effects of employment on the workers. In the pre-First World War years and during the war the Scottish Department of Health carried out a detailed investigation into chronic incapacity for work. Doctors working in the Clyde basin were asked to refer essential war workers thought to be nearing health break down, for convalescence. The experiment eventually took in the whole of the central belt and revealed a strong link between long hours of work and poor general health.[36]

However, the idea that a more interventionist attitude should be adopted regarding occupational health had a long history in the area, and such an approach was endorsed by the Department of Health for Scotland, Glasgow Corporation, and Glasgow's Public Health Authority. Glasgow's public health department was established in 1863, and over the next hundred years was involved with several important health initiatives: immunisation schemes; the establishment of smoke control areas; the eradication of unfit housing; the introduction of a family planning service; and a mass x-ray campaign. However, the department also adopted a pioneering approach to the question of occupational health, and was prepared at one point to fully incorporate occupational health within its jurisdiction. In the early 1950s the owners of a weaving mill in the East End of the city approached the department for help in tackling high absenteeism and a high accident rate amongst their 500 workers. The health officers found that poor air quality, bad lighting, and a lack of seats for the employees, were causal factors. Once these defects were rectified the accident and sickness rate was reduced dramatically. Moreover, a medical service was established for the factory with the co-operation of local GP's and this improved the health of the workforce even more. The public health department adopted a similar approach when it addressed the issue of poor health amongst the city's 2,400 cleansing department employees. Every employee was given a health check, and a job analysis of all the personnel revealed that many were being asked to perform tasks incompatible with their state of health and physique. Subsequently, several men were allocated less strenuous jobs. This, plus a crucial reduction in dust levels at work, reduced absenteeism, improved the general health and boosted the morale of the workers involved.

Glasgow Corporation had its own occupational health section responsible for conducting medical examinations of potential recruits to all the corporation's departments - except the police, fire, and transport departments which had their own medical officers. In the early 1950s this department also demonstrated its effectiveness in conducting occupational health research and acting upon its findings. The poor general health record and high absentee rate amongst the corporation's 42 sewermen, caused the department to closely investigate the nature of this work. The result of the investigation was that ventilation of the sewers was improved, washing and changing facilities were made available to the men, annual medical inspections were initiated, and service down the sewers was limited to 20 years. A similar approach was adopted by the Corporation during an investigation of Glasgow's fish market porters, when it was found that the high incidence of Weil's disease amongst the workers was caused by the handling of slimy fish boxes which had been soiled by rats.[37]

The success of these ventures convinced Glasgow's Medical Officer of Health in the early 1950s that there was a need for a proper occupational health service. Such a service he believed, could be effectively provided by a local health authority at no extra cost to the taxpayer, and that the benefits to society would be immense: 'If occupational health services were put into full operation throughout industry and succeeded in preventing widespread sickness, there might come a time when many of the hospitals could be closed down.'[38]

The results of Glasgow's pioneering occupational health experiments were conveyed to the aforementioned Dale committee - sitting at the time to examine the practicalities of setting up a national occupational health service. Although the committee refused to bow to the weight of evidence suggesting that an OHS should be established within the NHS, it did recommend that large local authorities should embark on empirical investigation along the lines of the Glasgow OHS initiatives. Unfortunately, though, the only public health authority in the UK to take up this challenge was Glasgow, where another pioneering occupational health experiment was initiated in 1953. The area chosen - Govan - contained over 8000 workers in 132 factories, along with 1200 shop assistants in 465 shops. These workers became the guinea pigs in what was to be the first large-scale occupational health experiment set up by a local authority. The investigation - organised by the Occupational Health Committee of the

BMA and the Society of Medical Officers of Health - found poor hygiene in the food factories, that the majority of engineering workplaces lacked any shower facilities, that cellulose paint spraying was being carried out without proper ventilation, that some of the wood factories had no proper dust control, and that most shops lacked separate washing facilities for the staff. One engineering firm was found to be referring 300 of its workers every year to Glasgow's Eye Infirmary - an excellent example of the NHS patching up the work wounded.[39] With the emphasis firmly placed on workers' health, many of these unhealthy and unsafe working practices were minimised. However, despite this effective demonstration of the benefits of medical intervention in the work environment, once again no other local authority followed Glasgow's lead.

The Govan experiment illustrated that small work units were much more susceptible to unhealthy working practices than larger industrial premises, and this was generally the case throughout the period. It was primarily to address this gap that the Nuffield Foundation sponsored the setting up of group occupational health schemes. The first such scheme came into being in Slough in 1947 where 52 firms agreed to pool their resources for the sake of workers' health. Five years later, at the end of Nuffield's funding period, there were 143 firms involved - although it should be noted that there were 300 firms in the immediate area. The scheme comprised a central clinic with accommodation for 65 patients and 20 out-patients; medical departments were set up in five of the largest firms; there were dressing stations, a mobile dressing station, and the monitoring of the health of the workers by meeting with their representatives every 2 months - all for the cost of 14/- (70 pence) per employee per year. During the ten years, which the Slough experiment ran, almost 25,000 preventative clinical examinations were undertaken by its medical staff.[40] A similar health service was established in Harlow in 1955 under Nuffield's funding initiative, and in 1960 the foundation pledged a further £250,000 towards the creation of more ventures. Consequently, a further five were set up throughout the country, including one in Dundee.

The Dundee scheme illustrates the difficulty of establishing voluntary occupational health services in a country, which already has a NHS. Nuffield stipulated that a minimum of 5,000 workers had to be involved before a centre could be opened. In 1962 the 14 employers in Dundee who had consented to taking part in the scheme could only muster 3,500. Consequently, the student health service at the University of Dundee agreed to take part in the scheme, and this brought the number up to over

5,000. Unlike Slough, there was no central clinic in Dundee. Instead, a team of nursing sisters in 4 minivans were each allocated a number of factories to visit on a regular basis. The nurses were encouraged to inspect their factories as much as possible and to become involved with preventative as well as curative care - 148 first aiders were trained by the service. A part-time medical officer was also engaged to tour each worksite, and this individual was also instructed to monitor unsafe working practices. The Dundee scheme cost each firm £2 per employee per year.[41]

However, although the Nuffield funded schemes met with some success, there were limitations. Firstly, all the schemes were set up in industrial estates where firms were in relatively close proximity to each other. The difficulty of setting up such a service in older industrial areas would have been much more problematic. Secondly, when Nuffield's funding initiative in this field ended, employers in other areas who tried to emulate the OHS schemes found that a general apathy and a lack of initial capital rendered this impossible. And thirdly, most of the initial schemes quickly folded when external funding was withdrawn. Consequently, although pointing the way ahead, the Nuffield experiments illustrated that private enterprise was unenthusiastic in becoming involved with providing occupational health services, and a principal reason for this was the existence of the NHS. Despite these important initiatives, then, occupational health coverage for small firms remained sparse throughout the period. A House of Lords Select Committee in the late 1980s drew attention to a need for such coverage amongst smaller firms. The Lords made three recommendations: smaller companies should be encouraged to buy the services of the occupational health departments of larger neighbouring businesses; that small firms approach local GP's and ask that an occupational health service be set up within their surgeries; or that smaller companies be encouraged to pool their resources and set up group OHS's along the lines of the Nuffield schemes.[42]

What is clear is that by the 1970s there was clear evidence that British occupational health provision was in need of urgent attention. Nuffield's initiatives and the various occupational health experiments had indicated that an interventionist preventative approach to health at the workplace could work. However, once again the state opted for laissez-faire.

The continuation of limited intervention

With the passage of the 1974 HSWA a number of industry-specific health and safety regulations were brought under one non-specific umbrella act - the main rationale being that individual laws relating to industrial processes could quickly become obsolete. General rules were laid down for employers and employees to follow. Employers were to 'ensure, so far as is reasonably practicable' the health and safety of their workers, and - 'so far as reasonably practicable' - provide a safe and healthy working environment with good welfare facilities.'[43] For their part, the workers were to 'take reasonable care' for their own and their fellow workers' health and safety, and co-operate - 'as far as possible' - with the employer to ensure that they [the employers] carried out their legislative responsibility.[44] This self-regulatory system was underpinned by two new agencies: the Health and Safety Executive (HSE), and the Health and Safety Commission (HSC). The HSE assumed responsibility for enforcing the HSWA, and was divided into several sections - such as factory inspectors, nuclear installation inspectors, etc. The HSC was a tripartite body made up of representatives from capital, labour, and government, and was designed to oversee all matters of health and safety and advise the government on such matters. At the same time the recently formed EMAS was brought under the auspices of the HSE.

How successful was the new system? A year after the HSWA was passed the Chief Inspector of Factories reported a drop in accident rates - although he took the opportunity to condemn the common practice amongst larger companies of delegating health and safety issues to semi-retired members of staff.[45] Further, statistics gathered six years after the inception of the HSWA also showed that fewer people were being killed or injured at work. This pattern, though, was reversed from 1981 onwards. From this period there was an increase in the number of small firms, and more larger companies began to depend on outside contractors.[46] Some employers fully embraced the responsibilities laid down by the 1974 Act. In 1988 Marks and Spencers employed over 200 doctors, 250 dentists, as well as chiropodists and nurses.[47] However, it was at the bottom end of the scale that voluntary participation in occupational health provision was most problematic. In 1976 the EMAS conducted a survey of over 3383 firms and found that the only OHS offered by 2,875 (85 per cent) of them was the provision of first aid. Only 84 of the companies surveyed employed medical and nursing staff.[48] A similar survey was conducted in 1993 and this showed little improvement regarding occupational health provision of smaller firms. Even more alarming was the revelation that although 81 per cent of private sector employers in the survey had heard of the HSE or the EMAS, just less than a third reported having any dealings with the agencies, such as a visit or a request for information.[49]

One of the Robens Committee's recommendations was that employers should have a statutory obligation to consult with their workers on occupational health and safety. The result of this was the Safety Representative and Safety Committees Regulations (SRSCR) of 1977. This provoked a flurry of activity and a survey conducted in 1977 found that over 80 per cent of the manufacturing establishments sampled had occupational health and safety committees in place.[50] The main flaw here, though, was that - contrary to the wishes of the Robens Committee - the new legislation only applied to unionised workers. Trade union membership in Britain reached a peak in 1979 when 63 per cent of male workers and 34 per cent of females were union members. However, this dropped steadily to reach a figure of 35 per cent and 30 per cent respectively by 1995.[51] This amounted to a sharp decline in the number of those covered by the 1977 legislation. Further, although employers were obliged to set up a safety committee if approached by at least two trade union safety representatives, the resultant committee could only serve as a forum for discussion and had no legal rights.

The SRSCR of 1977, then, did not usher in a new era of capital/labour collaboration over workplace health and safety. Its scope was limited by the fact that it excluded most of the British workforce - and the rise in the number of small firms in which trade unionism was poorly represented made this even worse. It also lacked any legislative backbone; and - like the whole HSWA itself - was based on the naive premise that capital and labour had an equal incentive to prioritise workplace health and safety.

Once again, then, the government's main control over unsafe working practices fell to the Factory Inspectorate. However, the notion that the FI could adequately protect workers from health risks was misplaced for three main reasons. Firstly, the coverage of the Inspectorate has always been inadequate. In 1971 in Scotland 50 inspectors were responsible for 25,000 industrial premises - this meant that on average an inspector made a visit to one of these establishments once every 4 years.[52] Throughout the UK the number of inspectors fell between 1979 and 1988, while the number of workplaces rose by 30 per cent. By 1986, therefore, there was a backlog of 10,000 overdue workplace visits throughout Britain.[53] The second shortfall of the factory inspection system was its lack of clout. It was common knowledge that the fines, which an inspector could impose, were modest, and this has remained so. In 1994-95 for example, the average fine imposed in the lower courts was just over £2,000. Moreover, up until 1996 no employer had ever been sent to prison for failing to comply with industrial health and safety legislation. Thirdly, the proficiency of the Inspectorate has also been called into question. Trade unionists have expressed a concern that many of the HSE personnel came from a management or university background, saw things in management terms, and were soft on employers.[54] Indeed, a Labour Research Department publication in 1975 conceded that this had been the case: 'the law has not been enforced by those whose duty it was to do so. It was the policy of the Factory Inspectorate to try to persuade employers to comply with legislation rather than to prosecute'.[55] There were certainly good grounds for this assumption when the Factory Inspectorate was implicated in the deaths of 40 Yorkshire asbestos factory workers in the late 1960s. Following an inquiry the Ombudsman found that factory inspectors responsible for the factory were guilty of negligence for not threatening the management with prosecution over the dangers of asbestos dust - a danger which they had been aware of for years.[56]

One of the main shortfalls was that the HSE - the body charged with ensuring the health of the workforce - and the Factory Inspectorate placed an emphasis on safety. Before being made part of the HSE in 1974 the Factory Inspectorate frequently issued safety publications, and organised lecture for shop stewards and trade union delegates on industrial safety. In the same way, the HSE initiated campaigns in the 1970s to ensure the safety of children in farms and building sites; published information on fork lift truck safety; and began a campaign in 1979 to encourage the breathalising of employees in certain industries. Even when William Simpson the chairman of the HSE - an ex iron moulder from Falkirk - visited Scott Lithgow's shipyard in 1977, his main concern was for the safety of welders working in confined spaces.[57] This was all highly commendable. However, such an emphasis ignored the fact that deaths from occupational disease in Britain were roughly 10 times higher than deaths from occupational accidents.[58] This heavy bias towards safety was directly acknowledged by the HSE in 1998 with the publication of its consultation document aimed at improving occupational health in the new millennium.[59]

Voluntary reporting of industrial disease has also been inadequate. In 1990 a labour force study found that over 2 million workers had an illness directly attributable to work - this accounted for 7 per cent of all GP consultations. This was much greater than the actual number of officially reported occupational illnesses. Even in Finland, where the reporting of occupational disease is more highly developed than in Britain, it is estimated that reporting underestimates the extent of industrially caused disease and injury by 3 to 5 times.[60] Recent legislation - the Reporting of Injuries, Diseases and Dangerous Occurrences Regulations 1995/96 - now legally compels employers to report cases of occupational disease. However, once again there is a tendency for under-reporting for several reasons. Firstly, there is no incentive for the employer to comply with the law, as notification would result in a visit from an inspector. Secondly, the employer is only under a legal obligation to report an industrial disease after he has been instructed to do so by a doctor. However, neither the patient nor the doctor may be aware that the illness is work related - and both may be unaware of the need to notify the employer.

The institutional structure upon which the HSWA stands has also proved to be shaky. Although the HSC was supposed to represent the state's involvement in occupational health - government representatives making up a third of its tripartite structure - tensions emerged between it and central government over the question of funding. In 1970-71 the government spent around £11 million on safety and health. The general secretary of the TUC estimated that because the health inspectorates were responsible for 1.25 million establishments, this amounted to the state spending £10 on each establishment per year towards its health and safety.[61] The funding situation was so bad in 1980 that the HSC published an article in the *Guardian* to express its concern at proposed funding cuts. Such cuts, it argued, would have meant an 8 per cent cut in its services, and a 20 per cent reduction in the number of doctors involved in occupational health work.[62] Moreover, eight years later the HSC actually commented on the shortfalls caused by the marginalisation of occupational health from the main body of the NHS. 'The separation of responsibility for occupational health from the NHS has inevitably led to a lower profile for occupational health issues within the NHS preventative, diagnostic, advisory, and treatment systems than might otherwise have been the case.'[63]

The inadequacy of the interface between OHS's and the NHS, alluded to by the HSC, has been highlighted in other studies.[64] A principal reason has been the lack of attention by the medical community specifically focused on work related bad health. Most GP's and medical students received no training in occupational health throughout the period. The Robens Committee acknowledged this, and recommended that this failure should be addressed. However, even by 1988 a House of Lords Select Committee noted that 'occupational health should be considered part of the primary care of patients, and GP's should take full account of the effects of occupation on health.'[65] This committee acknowledged that the relationship between primary health care and occupational health care was a slim one, and advocated that more use should be made of health centres as operational bases for the provision of area-based occupational health services.[66] However, nothing was done along these lines.[67] The difficulty of distinguishing occupational ill health from bad health, in which no work factors are involved, must be conceded. However, this difficulty has been compounded by the existence of professional boundaries. The majority of occupational health staff working in industry have no professional qualifications, and this lack of expertise is made worse by a polarisation of doctors and specialists into two separate professional camps.[68] On the one hand, GP's feared an encroachment of occupational health doctors into their own domain; while doctors specifically involved with occupational health concentrated on retaining this field as a separate medical discipline.[69]

The consequences of limited intervention: Asbestos

The limitations of the NHS in the sphere of occupational health are well demonstrated by reference to the experience of workers exposed to asbestos since World War Two. Asbestos is now killing more people in Britain than any other single industrial disease this century, and the sheer extent of this disaster illustrates three things. Firstly, the assumption that private capital could be entrusted with the responsibly of ensuring the health of the workforce was - and still is - misplaced. Secondly, that the focus of British health care, with its emphasis on cure and compensation, rather than prevention, has been misdirected. And thirdly, that the system of British occupational health coverage policed by the Factory Inspectorate, the HSE and the HSC has been inadequate, not least because of the emphasis these bodies place upon safety at work rather than health at work.

The major illnesses caused by exposure to asbestos are asbestosis, pleural plaques, pleural thickening, lung cancer, and mesothelioma. Asbestosis refers to scarring of the lungs by asbestos fibres and can take 15-30 years before any symptoms become apparent. The disease is progressive and incurable, causes pain and disablement, and may eventually lead to heart or lung failure. Thickening of the pleura - the membrane between the lungs and the rib cage - is also caused by the inhalation of asbestos dust, and results in progressive breathlessness. Pleural plaques are isolated thickened areas on the pleura and can be painful and debilitating - especially when another asbestos-related disease is present. By far the most serious is mesothelioma. This was, until fairly recently, a rare form of cancer, and is almost wholly related to asbestos. The disease can present up to 40 years after the victim's first exposure to asbestos, results in a high degree of pain, and normally kills the sufferer within a year of diagnosis. Between 1968 and 1991, 1,020 Scots have died of this condition.

The impact of asbestos on Clydeside has been catastrophic. The first companies manufacturing asbestos appeared in Glasgow in the 1870s and the industry proliferated thereafter. By 1900, there were 52 companies listed as 'asbestos manufacturers' in the Glasgow Post Office Directory.[70] The versatility of the material led to a massive proliferation in asbestos manufacture after World War One, and imports into the Clydeside region increased 30 fold between 1920 and 1967.[71] By the 1950s Clydeside companies were manufacturing a massive range of products from the raw asbestos shipped into Glasgow docks, including asbestos cement products (from Turner's factory in Clydebank), asbestos sheeting (from the Marinite factory in north Glasgow) and brake and clutch linings (from Ferodo, Glasgow). The material was extensively used on Clydeside in shipbuilding and engineering to cover and insulate pipes, boilers and electrical equipment (including wiring and electric motors). In the 1950s there were at least 20 thermal insulating companies operating on Clydeside working with asbestos in the shipyards. The biggest shipbuilders, such as John Brown's, had their own asbestos preparation sheds in situ in the yard. Some used the yards' air raid shelters left over from the war. Apart from those employed in asbestos manufacturing and the insulation trades occupational exposure included dockers, labourers and warehousemen at the point of entry at the port, carters and other transport workers, those in friction materials manufacture and electrical engineering, and construction workers. Tragically, a number of Scottish housewives also contracted asbestos-related diseases as a consequence of exposure to dust brought home on their husbands' work clothes.

The dust control regulations for asbestos developed from the early 1930s were targeted at asbestos manufacture. What was not realised, though, was that those also at risk were the workers who used the 'magic mineral' once it had been produced. Many workers had realised this for some time and the Home Office raised concerns about asbestosis amongst insulation workers in shipbuilding as early as 1945.[72] Voluntary measures implemented after the war proved to be ineffective in containing the asbestos hazard in shipbuilding. Public awareness was raised in the 1960s after new Shipbuilding Regulations (1960) incorporated legally enforceable preventative measures against the inhalation of asbestos dust for the first time. In 1962 a senior medical inspector of factories told Glasgow's Rotary Club of his fears concerning the dangers of asbestos, and commented that even a very short exposure to asbestos could result in health damage years after.[73] Joiners handling and cutting asbestos sheets aboard the new Cunard liner - destined to be known as the QE2 - in John Brown's shipyard, expressed alarm over risks to their health. This resulted in a visit by a trade union appointed doctor who assured the men that not all of the sheets they were handling were made of blue asbestos. At the same time, however, those employed to lag and insulate pipes with asbestos began to express their concerns.[74] This discontent resulted in a strike in June 1967 by 500 of Scotland's 700 insulating engineers - or laggers - over lack of protection against asbestos at work. According to the men there had been 53 cases of asbestosis in the Glasgow area alone since 1962, and 14 had already died of the disease. Frequently, laggers referred to the air so laden with asbestos dust that it was described as 'falling like snow'.[75] One of the main demands by the men was for a complete change of clothing so that any dangerous dust would not be taken from the workplace to their homes. They also demanded better washing facilities as opposed to the 'clean rags and pails of water' that they were expected to use. More importantly, they condemned the regular x-rays which they were subjected to as inadequate, and demanded a full medical examination. The strike was unofficial, and the trade union convinced the men to go back to work so that proper negotiations could begin with the employers.[76] The legacy for the Clydeside laggers was a particularly grim one. The asbestos-related disease registry compiled by the laggers branch of the TGWU in Glasgow listed 177 members suffering from some degree of disability, with 73 fatalities caused by asbestos between 1975 and 1981. The average age of death was 58 years.[77]

In the post-war period the use of asbestos was growing in construction because of its fire-resistant properties. Glasgow Corporation's Housing Department undertook to build high-rise multi-story housing where asbestos was used extensively. The Red Road flats in the north of the city (built 1961-1967) became notorious as the incubator of a cluster of asbestos-related disease. Here the joiners engaged in cutting and fitting the material earned the nickname 'white mice' because of their consistently dusty appearance. Surveys in the 1980s indicated death rates at between 10-33 per cent of those workers directly exposed to asbestos on the site. The average age of death was 51 years and 87 per cent of all deaths were due to asbestos-related cancers. The fact that a mobile occupational health unit had to be drafted in from Dundee to monitor the situation at Red Road provides an indication of the lack of local provision for industrial health in Glasgow at this time.[78]

From the war until the mid-1980s when the intense media attention surrounding asbestos became impossible to ignore, asbestos continued to be used extensively throughout Clydeside and beyond. However, over this same period medical knowledge of the dangers of asbestos was expanding. This, awareness though, was not effectively filtered down into the work environment, because the workplace was outwith the reach of national care. By 1991, when the sheer extent of the asbestos tragedy was clearly visible, the HSE's own mortality study of workers thought to have been most at risk from asbestos had revealed that 183 people in the survey group had died of mesothelioma since 1970. However, over the same period, the Mesothelioma register recorded over 10,000 deaths in the UK.[79] A large proportion of the latter deaths was historic, due to exposures prior to 1970. Nonetheless, the evidence still strongly indicates that in the 1960s and 1970s the focus of the HSE had been far too narrow, and that they had failed to pick up the wider health implications of industrial exposure to asbestos - amongst such diverse trades as plumbers, electricians, plasterers, welders, dockers, machine tool operators and the like.

Latterly, several legal measures have been put in place to protect workers from asbestos exposure. In 1983 the existing Asbestos Regulations were superseded by new regulations which made it a legal requirement that any worker working with asbestos insulation or asbestos coating must be medically examined before commencing employment with a company, and at a maximum of 2 year intervals thereafter. More recently, the Control of Asbestos at Work Regulations of 1987 finally acknowledged the extent of the problem in that any worker exposed to asbestos - not just in stripping or coating - should have regular medical checks. The importation of blue and brown asbestos into the UK was legally banned in 1984 and imports of chrysotile (white asbestos) banned in November 1999. For many, though, the regulations have come too late.

Our research project - funded by the Nuffield Foundation - investigated the social history of asbestos disease on Clydeside through oral history interviewing. What emerged from this study is that despite the existence of a Welfare State, most of the asbestos victims who responded to our questionnaire will finish their lives in relative poverty.[80] What is also interesting is that around half of our respondents stated that their GP's did not give them sufficient information (several deliberately) to assist them in their claims for benefit and compensation. More importantly, most interviewees remarked that their doctors did not immediately connect their work experiences with their ill health - asthma being wrongly diagnosed for asbestosis on three occasions. This further suggests that the general marginalisation of workplace health within the NHS has had serious consequences, and deserves further investigation. We also asked our respondents if they had ever had any experience with the HSE or the Factory Inspectorate. Hardly any of them had ever seen or been aware of a workplace visit by the HSE. A retired heating engineer had this to say regarding HSE inspections of building sites:

'We got a visit now and again but to me they were forewarned. I think so, because eh, when the site was getting tidied up, and all of a sudden the hard hats had tae be worn you know? So you knew there was somebody coming.'[81]

And a shipyard shop steward convenor also noted the limited role played by the HSE, and especially in relation to safety rather than health:

'It was more accidents, you know is the staging safe? Are you using proper ropes? Proper wires? They would check periodically, but you never heard anything about internal breathing or anything like that you know?'[82]

More importantly, it became apparent from the interviews we conducted that the system of trade union appointed safety representatives - set up following the 1974 HSWA - has tended, like the HSE and the Factory Inspectorate, to prioritise worker safety and not workers' health. However, despite the failings of the system it would be unfair to blame the unions for failing to take action over something about which they did not fully know the dangers; safety issues were, after all, much more immediate and could be more easily addressed than long-term health risks. What is inexcusable, though, is the fact that increasing medical knowledge was not immediately channelled into protecting workers from risk. The 30-year gap between a full realisation of the dangers of asbestos dust and the implementation of comprehensive protective safety measures in the late 1980s still needs to be explained. An engineer who was exposed to asbestos in the shipyards in the 1970s commented on the legacy of this neglect:

> They didn't even tell you to wear a scarf around your mouth. And, it must be stressed I know now - not so much back in the 1950s when I served my time with Barclay Curle, 'cause I'm not sure that they knew then that asbestos was a deadly substance. But by God they knew when I worked in Fairfields. It was known then to these people that asbestos was a deadly substance, and still they never gave us masks to wear and we were exposed to that stuff. Not even the laggers wore masks. So everybody that worked close to these guys, no matter what they were - be they electricians, marine engineers, laggers, or whatever - were exposed to that.[83]

Finally, it should also be noted that oral evidence from those exposed to asbestos at work on Clydeside illustrates that basic preventative measures such as the consistent use of respirators, dust suppression and health checks, were sometimes flouted by workers. There were several reasons for this: The workers were socialised into a stoical acceptance of poor health standards at work; they were unaware of the *extent* of the risks involved; they sometimes felt pressurised by the management; and they felt a need to cut corners in an effort to maximise their earnings.

Conclusion

The present government has recently launched an attack on social exclusion, and in 1997 Scotland's own Social Exclusion Network was set up. There are also high hopes that Scotland's new Parliament will focus more attention and resources on the issue of social exclusion. What is lamentable, though, is that the newly devolved Scottish Executive does not have any control over Scottish occupational health - which still remains with the bodies set up under the HSWA - for it is at the workplace that many health-related inequalities could be quickly addressed. It has been estimated that over the next 25 years a quarter of a million people will die in Britain because of exposure to asbestos at their work.[84] By far the majority of these individuals could be termed as belonging to the working class. Therefore, the notion that the working class has derived less benefit from national health care policy than other classes is difficult to challenge on the strength of this evidence. Many of these sufferers will also have spent most of their adult lives working for small companies in diverse work sites where occupational health care was non-existent, and where visits from the factory inspector were few and far between. The long latency period of their disease means that many of them were in contact with asbestos at work throughout the 50 years in which the NHS has been in existence. But all the NHS has done for them is provide palliative care long after the damage had been done. Sadly, this is a case in which the work wounded cannot be sent back into the field of battle.

Despite the importance of Britain's NHS, then, its continued emphasis on curative rather than preventative care means its impact as a social welfare measure has been blunted. The omission of an occupational health service reflects this emphasis on the curative. Over much of the 50 year period in which the NHS has been in existence, the medical profession, the trade union movement, and many workers themselves, have asked that occupational health be given much more attention. Despite this, occupational health has consistently been treated as a distant relative of mainstream health care - and we can only hope that the new consultation approach adopted by the HSE will address this. It is significant, however, that a new book detailing 50 years of the NHS - with a forward by the Prime Minister - makes no mention of the subject.[85] The NHS did not embrace and integrate occupational health and safety for a number of reasons; clashes of interest between ministries (especially Labour and Health); cost, in a period of spiralling health expenditure; and a prevailing sense by policy-makers that the NHS would be the panacea for all ills. This was in the face of concerted campaigns on the part of the trade unions to strengthen occupational health provision. The protective matrix offered by the state was further diluted by the disbanding of the government's occupational health research bureau in 1948 and flawed by the multiplicity of agencies with different methods and standards responsible for workplace inspection and policing - not to mention the widespread evasion of the legislation, and the ineffective penalties for factory crime. The onset of economic depression, the collapse of trade union power and deregulation from the late 1970s only made matters worse. The occupational health experiments conducted on Clydeside in the 1950s, and Nuffield's schemes in the 1960s clearly demonstrated the benefits of a preventative approach to occupational health. Had the state and/or local government taken the same interventionist approach, and had the overall attitude to industrial health been less skewed towards compensation and cure, then a great many people, now stricken with the worst industrial disease this century, would have been saved a painful, humiliating, and impoverished end.

Notes

1.	H. Wilson quoted in V. Navarro, *Class Struggle, the State and Medicine* (1978), p. xiii; M. Foot in R. Klein, *The Politics of the National Health Service* (New York, 1983), p.1.
2.	H. Jones, *Health and Society in Twentieth Century Britain* (1994), pp.177-182; D., Eva, and R., Oswald *Health and Safety at Work* (1981), pp. 88-89.
3.	J. A. Vaughan, 'The GP and Industrial Health', *Journal of the College of General Practitioners*, 26 (1960), p.13.
4.	See P.W.J. Bartrip and S.B. Burman *The Wounded Soldiers of Industry* (Oxford, 1983).
5.	See A.J. McIvor, 'Employers, the Government and Industrial Fatigue in Britain, 1890-1914', *British Journal of Industrial Medicine*, 1987, vol. 44; A. J. McIvor, 'Work and Health, 1880-1914', *Scottish Labour History Society Journal*, 24, (1989).
6.	HSC, *OHSs, the Way Ahead* (1977) p.2.
7.	J.A. Vaughan Jones, 'The GP and Industrial Health', *Journal of the College of General Practitioners*, 26 (1960), p.17.
8.	*Transactions of the Association of Industrial Medical Officers*, Oct. 1952, p.167.
9.	*Report of a Committee of Enquiry on Industrial Health Services, 1951* [Cmd.8170], p.5.
10.	See A.J. McIvor 'Manual work, technology, and industrial health 1918-1939', *Medical History*, 31, 2 April 1987, pp.160-189.
11.	*Report of the Committee on Safety and Health at Work 1970-1972*, p.632 - Henceforth Robens Committee.
12.	*Report of the Committee on Safety and Health at Work 1970-1972*, p.632 - Henceforth Robens Committee, Appendix D, p.27.
13.	J.A. Vaughn Jones, 'The GP in Industrial Health', *Journal of the College of General Practitioners*, 26 (1960), p.17.
14.	*Ministry of Health Department of Health for Scotland. A National Health Service 1944* [Cmd.6502].
15.	Transactions of AIMO, Oct. 1952, p.166.
16.	*Journal of College of General Practitioners*, 1, 141 (1958), p.144.
17.	R. Klein, *The Politics of the National Health Service*, (New York, 1983), p.1.
18.	*Glasgow Herald*, Leader, Feb. 27 1951, p.2.
19.	H. Jones, *Health and Society in Twentieth Century Britain* (1994), p.121.
20.	J.A. Vaughn Jones, 'The GP in Industrial Health', *Journal of the College of General Practitioners*, 26 (1960), p.18.
21.	Robens Committee, p. 555.

22.   *Committee of the Privy Council for Medical Research*, 1947, p.22. The Factory Inspectors' Reports in the 1930s also bear testimony to employers' 'minimalist' philosophy outwith a thin strand of avowedly 'welfarist' companies. Clearly, occupational health standards varied widely across the labour force, with wide differences in experience across the 'basic' and the 'new' industries in the 1930s.

23.   *Industrial Health Services Report 1951*, p.19.

24.   [Cmnd. 7664] 1949. The Gowers Committee recommended that OHSs should be extended to non-industrial enterprises too. *Glasgow Herald*, 27, Feb., 1951, p.4.

25.   See P. Weindling (ed.), *The Social History of Occupational Health* (1985), p.26.

26.   For a critique of the 'union failure' thesis in respect of occupational health see A. J. McIvor, 'State Intervention and Work Intensification' in A. Knotter, B. Altena and D. Damsma (eds.), *Labour, Social Policy, and the Welfare State* (Amsterdam, 1997), pp.134-136.

27.   *Transactions of AIMO*, Oct. 1952, pp.164-166.

28.   *Transactions of AIMO*, Oct. 1952, p.692.

29.   73rd Annual Report of the STUC, 1970, p. 128. Also, 76th Annual Report of the STUC, (1973), p.110.

30.   *Annual Report of the Chief Inspector of Factories 1958*, p. 52. [Cmnd. 811].

31.   Robens Committee, p.632.

32.   Robens Committee, p.690. *Glasgow Herald*, Dec. 20, 1960, p.4.

33.   *Report of the Royal Commission on Medical Education 1968* [Cmnd 3569].

34.   Robens Committee, p.691.

35.   76th Annual Report of the STUC, (1973), p.111.

36.   *Health Bulletin of Chief Medical Officer of the Department of Health for Scotland*, 3, 1, Dec. 1943, p.2.

37.   *Transactions of AIMA*, 2, Jan 1953, p.141.

38.   *Glasgow Herald*, April 15, 1952, p.3.

39.   *Glasgow Herald*, Jan. 14, 1954, p.6.

40.   *Transactions of AIMO*, 6, 8, (1956), p.153.

41.   *Transactions of AIMO*, 14, 66, (1964), pp.66-69. See also Robens Committee, evidence of Society of Occupational Medicine, pp.636-638.

42.   Editorial, 'OHSs for small workplaces' *Public Health*, 99 (1985), p.1.

43.   Eva & Oswald, *Health and Safety*, p.38.

44.   HSC Brochure *Health and Safety at Work Act, Advice to Employees.*

45.   *Glasgow Herald*, Dec. 4, 1975, p.7.

46.   H. Jones, *Health and Society in Twentieth Century Britain* (1994), p.152.

47.   S. Harvey, *Just an Occupational Hazard?* (1988), p.23.

48.   *Occupational Heath and Safety, the Way Ahead* (1977) HSC, p.7.

49.   K. Bunt, *Occupational Health Provision at Work* (1993), p.11.

50.   A. E. Glendol and R. T. Booth 'Worker participation in occupational health and safety in Britain' *International Labour Review*, 121, 4 (1982), p.403.

51.   C. Wrigley, *British Trade Unions 1945-1995*, (1997), p.29.

52.   *Glasgow Herald*, June 25, 1971, p.14.

53.   S. Harvey, *Just an Occupational Hazard?* (1988), p.19.

54.   Eva and Oswald, *Health and Safety*, p.53.

55.   *Labour Research Department Guide to the Health and Safety at Work Act* (1975), p.4.

56.   *Glasgow Herald*, March 30, 1976, p.4.

57.   *Glasgow Herald*, Sept. 27, 1977, p.8.
58.   S. Harvey, *Just an Occupational Hazard?* (1988), p.15.
59.   HSE, *Developing an occupational health strategy for Great Britain* (1998).
60.   Snashall, p.1.
61.   C. Wrigley, *British Trade Unions 1945-1995,* (1997), p.202.
62.   Eva & Oswald, *Health and Safety*, p.55. Things haven't changed much. One of the recommendations for curbing the high death toll caused through asbestos exposure was for the HSE to supply a cheap face mask to all those involved. However, the HSE have recently stated that it does not have the money for such an initiative, and that employers should be made to provide such protection. BBC Radio 4 programme 'Too Little Too Late' 15 Oct. 1998.
63.   HSC, (1988), p.22.
64.   See J. McEwan et al, 'The interface between OHSs and the National Health Service', *Public Health*, 96 (1982), pp.155-163.
65.   Quoted in S. Harvey, *Just an Occupational Hazard?* (1988), p.26.
66.   Gregson Report (1984) A report of a sub-committee of the House of Lords Select Committee for Science and Technology on Occupational Health and Hygiene HMSO.
67.   Indeed, in 1992 a HSE survey recommended that training in occupational health should be included in the course curriculum of health practice nurses. See N. Griffin, *Occupational health advice as part of primary health care nursing* HMSO (1992), p.2.
68.   B. Jacobson *et al, The Nation's Health* (1991).
69.   S. Harvey, *Just an Occupational Hazard?* (1998), p.11.
70.   *Post Office Directory of Glasgow*, 1900-1901.
71.   G. H. Roberts, Necropsy studies of asbestos bodies in Glasgow and a clinico-pathological study of pleural mesotheleoma. Medical Thesis, University of Wales (1968), p.80.
72.   Letter, A.W. Garrett, Chief Inspector of Factories, to J.W. Roberts (asbestos manufacturers) Leeds, August 1945 (Turner and Newall Archive, Clyde Action on Asbestos, Glasgow)
73.   *Glasgow Herald*, 31 Jan. 1962, p.6.
74.   *Glasgow Herald*, 24 Feb. 1967, p.24.
75.   Social History of Asbestos Project, Scottish Oral History Centre, University of Strathclyde. Interviewees A2; A3; A18.
76.   *Glasgow Herald*, 13 June 1967, p.11.
77.   TGWU, Insulating Engineers 7/162 Branch, Confirmed Asbestosis Cases Register, 1975-1981.
78.   T. Gorman, 'The Continuing Use of Asbestos in Buildings', Paper to the 17th Proceedings of the BISS, Glasgow 1995, pp.32-4; *Scottish Daily Express*, 27 March 1984; Greater Glasgow Health Board, Occupational Health Service, 'Red Road Construction Workers Survey, 1985-6' (Unpublished Report, May 1986). At 32 storeys the Red Road flats were the highest in Europe.
79.   HSE, *Occupational Health Decennial Supplement* (1995), sec. 9.1
80.   See R. Johnston and A. McIvor, 'Pushed into social exclusion: Asbestos-related disability and relative poverty on Clydeside', *Scottish Affairs*, forthcoming Spring 2000. Also, R. Johnston and A. McIvor, *A Lethal Business: Asbestos on the Clyde*, (Tuckwell Press, forthcoming 2000).

81.   Social History of Asbestos Project, Scottish Oral History Centre, University of Strathclyde, Interviewee A7.
82.   Social History of Asbestos Project, Scottish Oral History Centre, University of Strathclyde, Interviewee A9.
83.   Social History of Asbestos Project, Scottish Oral History Centre, University of Strathclyde, Interviewee A8.
84.   Peto *et al*, 'Continuing increase in Mesothelioma mortality in Britain', *The Lancet*, Vol. 345, March 4, 1995, pp.535-539.
85.   G. Rivett, *From Cradle to Grave 50 Years of the National Health Service* (London, 1998).

7. Scotland, Social Justice, Health and Inequality

HUGH McLACHLAN

Introduction

It is said in the Green Paper on *Working Together for a Healthier Scotland* that: 'For 50 years, the NHS has helped people who fall sick'.[1] What the document advocates is: '... a restructuring of the National Health Service as a public health organisation with health improvement as its main aim'.[2]

It is said too that:

'A fresh approach is necessary - a public health strategy which addresses the root causes of our health problems.... The need is to ensure that each strand of policy and every new initiative, is taken forward within a coherent framework, so that health gain is maximised. Above all, we need to attack the inequalities which scar our health record.'[3]

These and many of the recent claims which have been made concerning health policy in and for Scotland - see, in particular, *The Possible Scot*[4] - can be better understood and evaluated by relating them to the Report of the Commission on Social Justice.[5]

According to Tony Blair: 'John Smith's anger at the state of Britain today led him to establish the Commission on Social Justice. Its report will inform Labour's policy making and provide the basis for a vital national debate about the future of work and welfare. It is essential reading for everyone who wants a new way forward for our country.'

The Report, to which the Prime Minister refers and on the blurb of which his comment appears is over four hundred pages long.[6] It is, arguably, the most interesting, comprehensive and challenging work of its sort since the Beveridge Report of 1942 on Social Insurance and Allied Services. According to the Report, the notion of 'social justice' can be defined in terms of a hierarchy of four ideas. They are these.

106

(1) First of all there is: '... the belief that the foundation of a free society is the equal worth of all citizens, expressed most basically in political and civil liberties, equal rights before the law, and so on'.[7]

(2) Secondly, there is: '... the argument that everyone is entitled, as a right of citizenship, to be able to meet their basic needs for income, shelter and other necessities. Basic needs can be met by providing resources for services, or helping people acquire them: either way, the ability to meet basic needs is the foundation of a substantive commitment to the equal worth of all citizens'.[8]

(3) Thirdly, according to the Report: '... self respect and equal citizenship demand more than the meeting of basic needs: they demand opportunities and life chances. That is why we are concerned with the primary distribution of opportunity as well as its redistribution'.[9]

(4) Fourthly, it is said that: '... to achieve the first three conditions of social justice, we must recognise that although not all inequalities are unjust (a qualified doctor should be paid more than a medical student), unjust inequalities should be reduced and where possible eliminated'.[10]

The Report and the Two Different Policy Aims

According to the Report:

'Discussion about health policy in the United Kingdom usually starts and ends with the National Health Service. We have taken a much wider view of the fundamental questions that our society needs to resolve. The first issue we address is how best to promote good health and reduce health inequalities.'[11]

The Report says:

'... it is essential that we start with the goal of improving health and reducing health inequalities - in other words, health gain - rather than allowing health policy to be dominated by the treatment of illness.'[12]

There are deceptively profound questions raised here. Should the state try to promote health? If it should do so, on what grounds should it? Should the state try to reduce health inequalities? If it should do so, on what grounds should it? If there is a conflict between the promotion of health and the reduction of health inequalities which of the two goals should be preferred? On what grounds should it be preferred?

What is called in the Report 'the first issue' actually comprises two issues. On the one hand, some steps - perhaps most or even all steps - to promote good health might increase health inequalities. For instance, health education schemes, if they have any beneficial effects at all, typically influence different people and different categories of people differently. On the other hand, some steps to reduce health inequalities might well not promote good health and might even do the opposite. For instance, to make the healthier less healthy will not necessarily improve the health of the less healthy. A reduction in, say, the inequalities of wealth holding could lead to a reduction in health inequalities without leading to an increase in the general level of health. Again, if the lifestyles of the 'working' and 'middle' classes, as conventionally conceived, were to become more similar, then health inequalities might decrease and the general level of health might decline in Britain depending on whether or not working or middle class patterns of, for instance, smoking and consuming fresh fruit and vegetables became the norms. If, say, the behaviour and circumstances of men and women become more similar, their health might become more equal but, overall, less good.

Justice, Health Care and the Promotion of Health

The Report implies and suggests that the state should, as a matter of justice (or social justice) promote health. This is implausible (although it should, perhaps, do so on other grounds such as, say, that of the promotion of individual freedom and autonomy or, say, that of the general utilitarian ground of increasing happiness or - better still - that of the non-ethical ground of improving economic efficiency).

The claim is made that we have a right to health. It says in the Report that:

> 'The right of equal access to health care should be part of a broader vision of social rights. If citizens are to enjoy a 'right to health', the right to health treatment and care must be seen as fundamental. The right to good health cannot in general be treated as a legal right; it is a moral and social right, to be realised through political action.'[13]

> 'Now, there are important distinctions between health care and health in relation to public policy, justice and rights. For instance, health care is something which individual people and public and private agencies can sometimes provide for other people. Health is not. Some of the factors

which can effect health can sometimes be provided but that is another matter.'

Le Grand takes a different view of the matter.[14] He writes:

'... it could be argued [that] health care is amenable to policies concerned with promoting equity in a way that health is not. Therefore, it makes more sense to talk of the equity or otherwise of the distribution of health care than of the distribution of health. But this is not very compelling. Although in one sense it is true that it is impossible to redistribute health, this does not mean that the distribution of health is insensitive to public policy. For it is obviously possible to influence by policy many of the factors that affect health, such as nutrition, housing and work conditions, and, of course, medical care itself.'[15]

As a university lecturer, I am responsible for marking students' essays and examination scripts. I have a duty to mark them impartially, accurately and equitably. It would not be true to say that I am obliged to treat my students equally in all respects: often different essays and different exam scripts should get different marks. The distribution of the essay and examination marks of my students, given the quality of the essays and examination scripts, is my responsibility. The distribution of health and happiness among my students is not at all my responsibility even although the distribution of essay and examination marks is among the factors which can affect student happiness and health. I have duties directly concerning the essay and examination marks of my students but not, in the same way concerning their happiness or health. Similarly, I think that there is a difference between talking about justice with regard to the distribution of (some) health care and talking about justice with regard to the distribution of health. While the state and governments can affect both, it and they are responsible only for the former.

The state in the UK is responsible, by virtue of the existence of the NHS, for the distribution of some health care. It would be wrong to say that all British citizens are entitled to an equal share of such health care or even to say that they should have 'equal access' to it. I live in Elderslie, Renfrewshire and do not drive a motor car. I do not have a share of, say, the M20 nor access to it equal to that of residents of London. No injustice, however, results from nor is contained in these facts. No one, whether sick or well has a right to treatment from the NHS We have, rather, a right to have our claims to treatment considered impartially. This is another way of saying that the relevant agents and agencies of the NHS have a duty not to refuse us on irrelevant grounds, refuse us though they might and may. That is what that and all that justice requires in relation to health care and public policy or so I would suggest.

If individual A is given a heart transplant by the NHS and individual B is not - unequal treatment is an essential feature of the NHS and, indeed, of all publicly provided services - then individual B might reasonably ask for a justification of this inequality. The NHS as an agency of the state should, by considering individual cases impartially, treat individual people differently - i.e. unequally - but justifiably so. 'There was only one heart available and we had to toss a coin. You lost.' That might well serve as a justification whether or not it would satisfy B.

Let us suppose that, prior to the heart transplant, A and B were equally unhealthy and far less healthy than C and D. Now, it might well be the case that A or B or both of them blame the state, to an extent, for their heart problems. Perhaps there is even some justification for their view. Perhaps they worked in the public sector and were unfairly harassed by their bosses. Perhaps the state has a duty to not avoidably make people ill. However, this would not the same as saying that the state has a duty to give people health and that, correspondingly, they have a right to health. If Kant is correct in saying that ought implies can, it would appear not to make sense to say that the state ought to provide us with health since health in other people (as opposed, sometimes, to ill health and death) is not producible at will (by the state nor by anyone nor anything else). If no one or nothing has a duty to provide A or B or you or me with health, then how could we be said to have a right to health?

If we do not have a right to health, then it does not seem that, in the name of justice, the state should promote health. Perhaps, nonetheless, the state should try to promote health. After all, one might say. for instance, that governments should do what they can reasonably can to try to promote high levels of employment even if A and B and you and I do not have a right to a job in the sense, say, that we have a right not to be killed or a right to a fair trial if we are accused of a crime.[16]

As we have seen, it says in the Report that: 'The right to good health cannot in general be treated as a legal right; it is a moral and social right, to be realised through political action.'[17] There is, of course, no legal right to health. If any Parliament were stupid enough to pass legislation which granted people a legal right to health, then, it would be mere words: it would not be a right which the state could have the power to honour.

Since no agent nor agency could have the power to honour it - and, perhaps, for other reasons as well - to call it 'a moral and social right' seems to me either to be meaningless or false.

The authors of the Report might be asked to clarify and elaborate upon what they mean by their very curious claim that there is a 'moral and social right' to health. After all, political action might result in the production of novel legal rights (whether they are worth having or not) or in particular outcomes (whether or not the participants had a moral or legal right to them) but how political action could create novel moral rights is, to say the very least, obscure. And, if a 'social' right is something other than a legal or a moral right, what sort of thing is it?

Justice and the Reduction of Inequalities in Health

Let us turn to the second issue, that of health inequalities. According to the Report: 'It is essential that [the] government sets clear goals for reducing health inequalities.'[18] Why it should be thought essential to set clear goals is not made clear. That, if it can do so, the government should try to reduce health inequalities is not shown either. The Report continues:

> 'In Merseyside, local health experts have proposed that by the year 2000 infant mortality rates and low birth rates in the most disadvantaged local area should be raised to those of the best-off area. Infant mortality rates are an important reflection of broader health inequalities, and we would like to see the British government commit itself to the goal of steadily cutting infant mortality and morbidity rates in the bottom social classes until the present gap is eliminated. These goals should be accompanied by clear strategies, so that all those responsible for other areas of policy know the contribution which they are expected to make to promoting better health; and progress towards the goals should be monitored and published.'[19]

It would be good if the infant mortality rates in the poorest area of Liverpool were to be reduced. What if they were to be reduced and, at the same time, the infant mortality rates of the best-off area were also to be reduced? Would that not be better still, even if health inequalities were not reduced? Why the stress on reducing inequalities? If the government is to be set clear - or, perhaps more usefully, vague - goals concerning health, why should they not relate to the promotion of good health and the reduction in ill-health no matter whether or not health inequalities are

increased or reduced? That, say, infant mortality rates for social category X
be the same as infant mortality rates for social category Y does not seem to
me to be a profoundly important policy aim no matter what 'X' and 'Y'
happen to stand for.

Apart from any other considerations, the distribution of health is
not a 'zero-sum game'. If, say, I own more land now than I did ten years
ago, you might think that my increased landholding must correspond to the
decreased land-holding of some other person or agency: there is only so
much land available to be parcelled off. If, however, I am healthier now
than I was ten years ago, it would be absurd to imagine that my increase in
healthiness was at the expense of someone else's corresponding decrease.
Indeed, my conspicuous increased healthiness and happiness may have had
on some benevolent and sympathetic people the effect of increasing theirs.

The Report says: 'Our aim is not to eliminate all health differences,
for that would be impossible, but rather to reduce or eliminate those that
result from factors which are both avoidable and unfair.'[20] This would seem
to be an attempted application of the notion that justice requires: '... that we
reduce and where possible eliminate unjustified inequalities.'[21] There is a
difference between eliminating our own avoidable actions and acting to
eliminate other phenomena which were not, or not solely, the consequences
of our actions and were not our responsibility.

Justice requires of us that, in some spheres of our actions, we treat
people equally unless there is a justification for our treating people
differently and that, where there is a justification for treating them
differently, we treat them differently. This is not the same as saying that:
'we are required to reduce and where possible eliminate unjustified
inequalities.' Not all inequality is our business nor responsibility. Not all
inequality is the business nor the responsibility of the state.

One might say that, in the name of justice, governments are
required to justify or cease their unequal treatment of people. They are not,
however, so required to justify or remove general inequalities such as, for
instance, inequalities of happiness, wealth or health.

Note also this complication: sometimes when an inequality is
unjustified it is not possible to remove it without acting unjustly.
Sometimes, avoidable and unjust and/or unfair inequalities can be avoided
by - and sometimes, perhaps, only by - the production of other (avoidable
and) unjust and/or unfair actions. For instance, adultery can be unfair and
unjust but so too can be some of the policies, for instance, forced female
circumcision and capital punishment, which can reduce its occurrence.

Women in Britain live on average longer than men. Is this fair? Is it unfair? I do not know. (Perhaps it is neither fair nor unfair: neither just nor unjust.) I most certainly do not think that public policy should be geared towards the elimination of this gender and health inequality. It would be possible to eliminate this inequality. For instance, the SAS could be employed to kill a sufficient number of women such that, on average, the life expectancy of men and women in Britain became the same. Not only would these means be unacceptable but so too would be the end of such a policy.

Suppose that it became possible to introduce some costless policy measure which had one and only one effect: that of increasing, on average, female life expectancy in Britain. I would be very much in favour of adopting this policy. It would lead to even greater inequality in relation to life expectancy but so what?

If there were a similar policy measure whose sole effect was an increase in the life expectancy of, say, middle class people, or of white people or of black people or of male, middle class, white people then I think that I would similarly be in favour of it. Why not? Equality for the sake of equality seems to me to be an absurd principle in the context of the average health of different social groups.

The Report contends that:

> 'This country is scarred by health inequalities. The poorest and least powerful members of our society are ill more often and die younger. Along with the gap between rich and poor, the gap between healthy and unhealthy has grown wider in the last decade, a direct result of more unemployment, more poverty, more stress and greater social inequality itself. The health gap between different social classes, different regions and different communities is not inevitable and is simply unacceptable.'[22]

If, on average, people who are poor are more likely to suffer from ill health and to die younger than people who are rich, then - whether or not it might be a good idea to try to install laws and public policies to alter the situation - the situation is not necessary an injustice nor the result of one. Those individuals who suffer from ill health and those individuals who die relatively young are not necessarily being deprived of the enjoyment of a right. Who or what has a duty to ensure that these particular individuals do not have an unusually short life span? Who or what has a duty to ensure that these particular individuals are not more unhealthy than richer people tend to be? Who or what has any other related obligation concerning the health and life span of these particular people?

It says in the executive summary of *The Possible Scot*:

> 'Average life expectancy in Scotland ranks with the former German Democratic Republic ... Many Scots fail to realise their own desired potential because of poverty and disease ... The challenge will be to ensure that reaching one's potential is not the preserve of the affluent but the birthright of all.'[23]

The reaching of one's potential is neither the preserve of the affluent nor the birthright of anyone. It is not a right in the sense that, say, we have a right to life in that all other people and agencies have a duty not wantonly to kill us. No one nor agency has a duty to ensure that you or I or any one else lives for a particular length of time and/or enjoys a particular level of health. Had we been born in, say, Japan rather than Scotland or in Scotland but of richer parents, then we might have had a greater chance of better health and a longer life than we have but it does not follow from this that our birthright to fulfil our potential has been denied us. There is no such birthright. Had we been born in Scotland in the nineteenth century rather than in Scotland in the twentieth then our life expectancy would have been lower than it is: yet, if we were born in Scotland in the twentieth century, that was a matter of luck rather than of right.

Some people, when they think that other particular people are, say, healthy and prosperous can, through humanitarian empathy gain pleasure from the thought. Some people, through envy, can be distressed by it. As a general thing, the envy should be disapproved of and should not be pandered to. However, sometimes, particularly when they are visible and extreme, inequalities can sometimes cause such distress that, in the interests of social harmony, it is justifiable to have public policies geared towards their reduction. Notice, however, that here such policies, when they are justified, are not justified on the grounds of justice but, rather, on other grounds and, sometimes justified despite the fact that the policies concerned are very unjust ones.

Politics is not reducible to ethics nor ethics to justice. For instance, 'affirmative action' programmes, by trying to produce equality of outcomes with regard to particular social categories of people, often - and perhaps even necessarily - deny individual people, as individual people, the impartial consideration which justice - and so-called 'equality of opportunity' - implies. How can one be both, say, gender vigilant and gender blind? However, such 'affirmative action' programmes, even if unjust, might sometimes be justifiable in terms of their consequences. (Of course, rather than producing social harmony, such programmes can themselves be socially divisive: 'positive discrimination' for X is often thought to be - and often is - straight-forward discrimination against Y.)

It is possible that, even if they are not justified on the grounds of justice, policies aimed at reducing inequalities of health might be justified on other grounds. However, it is not clear how such a justification could be presented. As a matter of fact, in contemporary Scotland and the contemporary UK, although some other inequalities might be, inequalities of health are not socially divisive. We might covet, say, our neighbour's house or, more likely, the houses of people who stay in better neighbourhoods than we do ourselves, but we are not in general envious of other people's health. One reason for this might be that while we might buy, steal or, one some other basis, acquire our neighbour's house, we cannot acquire his health: health is non-transferable. Among the various other reasons is that, in general, people do not tend to think of themselves as having, say, a life expectancy which is different from other people around them who are members of different social categories from them. Relative death rates are, in any case, not widely known nor highly visible.

The Promotion of Happiness and the Reduction of Happiness Inequalities.

The two issues of health promotion and the reduction of health inequalities are, in my view, curious ones for any government or state to address. For instance, suppose that one were to say: Discussion about happiness in the United Kingdom usually starts and ends with such-and-such. We have taken a much wider view of the fundamental questions that our society needs to resolve. The first issue we address is how best to promote happiness and reduce happiness inequalities. The promotion of happiness is one aim and the reduction of happiness inequalities is another. They might well be conflicting aims. Should they be aims of state policy at all?

The causes of happiness, it seems to me, are so varied and complex that it might, perhaps, be best for governments not to be too concerned with its promotion or control, particularly since governments have, as it is, a plethora of tasks to attend to. Furthermore, if citizens choose actions which lead to their own unhappiness, it is not at all clear what business of governments this is. Governments might, perhaps, more reasonably and modestly try to reduce some of the causes of misery and, say, try to disseminate information which, if people choose to act upon it might make them happier. If some people are happier than others, then what business of or source of concern to governments is this? It was not their doing: it is not their responsibility. In any case, one might suggest, 'happiness' is too difficult to define and, for the purposes of public policy objectives, far too vague a notion to be of much, if any, practical use.

What was said here about happiness might be said about health. For instance, one might ask: what does 'health' mean? In *The Possible Scot*, it is noted that the death rate is higher in Scotland than in Britain as a whole. This is the basis given for the claim that 'Scotland has a depressingly poor health record.'[24] That the death rate is a good indication of the health of a group of people is an assertion which is very commonly made, but it is not one which is self-evidently true. Not all deaths are the result of ill health. For instance, suicide and accidents can cause death. Some seemingly healthy people die and it is dogmatism to say that they must have been unhealthy, despite appearances, otherwise they would still be living. Contrariwise, some manifestly unhealthy people continue, stubbornly, to live.

Donald Dewar says in the preface to Working for a Healthier Scotland:'

> Age at death is a crude measure, if a hard test, of our health progress. In reality, good health is the basis for happy childhood, achievement in middle years and independence in old age. It is not just death but pain, depression, fear and disablement that put a limit on lives, and impose social and economic burdens.[25]

It is true to say that it is not merely death which limits our lives and imposes social and economic burdens but it is equally true to say that it is not merely ill health which does so. Similarly, ill health is not the only cause of unhappiness in childhood and so forth; health is not the only factor which can be productive of its opposite. Consequently, the platitudes of Scotland's First Minister do not help here to bring us any closer to a workable definition of 'health'.

The following quote from the Green Paper is not much help either: 'Good health is more than the absence of disease. It has to do with the way we live, the quality of our life and our environment.'[26]

Age at death might or might not be a measure of health progress. In order to know whether or not it is, we would require some other criterion of health against which to plot the death rate. How else could we judge how useful a measure of health progress the death rate is? No such criterion of 'health' has, to my knowledge been suggested. To say, in the famous words of the WHO that 'health' is: 'a state of complete physical, mental and social well-being and not merely the absence of disease or infirmity' is like mouthing hollow encouragement, in the manner of a diffident audience at a poorly performed pantomime - oh, yes it is! - rather than giving practical assistance in a definitional task.

One might say too that not everything that could be done to increase happiness and/or improve health ought to be done and that not everything, which ought to be done, ought to be done for the sake of justice.

Suppose that the health (and/or the happiness) of people in general in Britain would be improved and ill health (and/or unhappiness) reduced if, say, smoking tobacco, drinking alcohol, and worrying were eliminated and if every one in Britain took frequent, vigorous exercise and had a sparse but nutritious diet. I am not saying that such a regime would lead to an improvement in health (and/or happiness), but suppose that it would. Would any and all measure which would or might produce it be justified? Surely not. Suppose that people were prevented from drinking alcohol and smoking tobacco by the illegalisation of the sale of those substances and by the severe and public corporal punishment of those who were discovered to have consumed them and that the health of the population improved. Would this improvement justify the illegalisation of the trade and the painful punishment of the criminals thereby created? Not in my view.

Marijuana, dissolved, somehow, independently of the knowledge and wishes of consumers in the public water supply might lead to an improvement in general health through a general reduction in anxiety. Would such a policy be justified? I think not.

Perhaps a health education policy which presented people with knowledge concerning smoking, worrying, drinking, exercise, nutrition and health and allowed them to make informed choices might be a justifiable means to the promotion of good health and the reduction of ill-health. There again, some such policies might not be justifiable depending on how reasonably the relevant 'knowledge' is presented and on how effective and how costly they happen to be. Information concerning, say, exercise and diet can be presented in such a po-faced way that it has little of its intended effect and perhaps even a counter effect. Persuasion, whether rational or not, is not always easy nor cheap.

Health and Holistic Government

It says in the Report that:

> Since good health is the result of factors that are almost entirely outside
> the control of the NHS, the goal of improving people's health will be
> served by spending outside and not only within the NHS, while the
> balance of NHS resources needs to be shifted further towards prevention
> rather than treatment. Spending a larger proportion of national income on
> the treatment of ill health does not necessarily improve a nation's health.[27]

This is not at all convincing. It might well be true to say that the
goal of improving health will be attained more efficiently by spending
money on something other than the treatment of illness but it does not
follow from this that improving health is a preferable goal to the treatment
of illness. (And what does such apparent hard-nosed economic efficiency
have to do with the notion that the promotion of health and the provision of
health care pertain to social justice?) Spending money on, say, roads, or
defence or on foreign aid will not necessarily improve a nation's health.
That is not in itself much of a reason against spending money on roads,
defence or foreign aid.

Even if the promotion of health is a general aim of public policy, it
is not the only one nor, by any means, the most important one. For instance,
suppose that you have toothache and/or a broken leg. You want the pain to
cease soon. It might well be that the treatment you receive has no effect on
your life expectancy and hence, as these things are measured, has no
beneficial effect on the 'health' of the nation. Little will that concern you so
long as the treatment rids you of the pain.

Good health is the result of factors which are beyond the control of
the NHS However, it does not follow that spending public money outwith
the NHS will have the effect of improving the health of the citizenry. Even
if it would do, such spending and the policies they involve might not be
justifiable. It all depends. Even if spending a larger proportion of national
income on the treatment of ill health does not improve the health of the
citizenry, it might still be a good idea to do so. It might, for instance,
increase their happiness or, at least, lessen their unhappiness.

According to the Report:

The new emphasis that we want to see on health promotion will require national and local government to take a fundamentally new approach to health. Instead of health being viewed as the concern only of the Department of Health and the regional and local health authorities, it should be integrated into the work of every department.[28]

On the one hand, this might sound like sensible 'joined-up' government. One the other hand, one must wonder whether governmental Departments have shown themselves to be so effective in the past that we can reasonably and confidently expect them comfortably and successfully to take on such an additional massive task.

Should they take on such a task? No one particular government department could cope with the goal of improving happiness, given all the possible causes of it. It does not follow from this that it would necessarily be a goal idea for all government departments to have a go at promoting it. The same might be said about health. And: why health? Why should health be elevated to such a position in public policy priorities? Would not, say, happiness, be a more reasonable (or less unreasonable) spectre to chase if one were to think that public policies should be particularly primed for the capture of a favoured quarry?

It says in *The Possible Scot* that:

'... if the determinants of health are multiple and interactive, then policy making must have these qualities. We need government machinery which is capable of comprehending the whole system, as a system, rather than its constituent parts: we need holistic government.'[29]

Again, it says that: 'If the determinants of health are multiple and interactive, policy making must not be fragmented but holistic. The argument for holistic government is thus inescapable.'[30]

The argument for 'holistic government' can be resisted. If the determinant of, say, happiness are multiple and interactive, it does not follow that public happiness policy must have these features. Perhaps there should be no public happiness policy nor policies. Perhaps there should be no 'holistic' government nor policies pertaining to health of the sort envisaged in *The Possible Scot*. The obvious danger of such a 'holistic' approach is that it encourages a monomaniacal approach to public policy. 'Health; health; health' as a slogan is no more attractive nor plausible nor wise than, say: 'Education; education; education' nor: 'Defence; defence;

defence'. Furthermore, the question arises of whether one wants to live under such a busy and fussy sort of government as that envisaged here.

Can Health Inequalities be Eliminated?

Are health inequalities inevitable? Perhaps they are; perhaps they are not. Perhaps even if we can, by design, remove some particular sort of health inequality, other ones will remain and other, perhaps unpredicted and unintended, ones might emerge. When we eliminate some avoidable inequalities, we can create other ones which might be no less unjust and/or unfair and which are not merely avoidable but would have been avoided if we had not eliminated the former inequalities. Whether or not particular health inequalities are inevitable, government will make it, in general, less pleasant or less healthy to be rich than to be poor.

Conclusion

In *The Possible Scot*, it says: 'We now have a great opportunity to face the challenge implicit in Scotland's poor health performance and to adopt a fresh approach to raising Scotland's health status.'[31]
     It continues:

> 'The cross-departmental commitment to the Green Paper within the Scottish Office suggests the beginnings of a style of government that we believe should be further developed and become the hallmark of the Scottish Parliament. If this approach can be developed, the potential impact of policy on health outcomes is enormous.'[32]

Scotland, compared with Britain as a whole and other similarly advanced countries has a high death rate. It is not thereby established that it has a poor health performance compared to them although it might have.
     Whether or not Scotland has a relatively low standard of health, it has not been established that a fresh approach to health policy is required nor that a three pronged strategy based upon: the promotion of health; an attack on health inequalities; and holistic health orientated government would be a wise one to adopt. The arguments which have been put forward in this regard concerning 'social justice', in particular, are unconvincing.
     The hierarchy of four ideas which are said to define 'social justice' and which were listed in the introductory section are all contestable. In particular, the relationship suggested in the Report between needs - whether

basic or not - and justice is highly dubious. For instance, I might need, say, oxygen and sex but it does not follow from that that the state or some other body or person is obliged to provide them for me nor that I am necessarily a victim of injustice if I do not receive them. We all need to be alive (and, to some extent, healthy) in order to be able to do anything at all yet, manifestly, although we have a right not to be killed unlawfully, we do not have a right not to die. Death is not in itself an injustice and neither, necessarily, is ill health.

Furthermore, there is more to politics than ethics and more to ethics than justice. Justice is a virtue but it is not the only one and it can conflict with other ones. A public library system, for instance, which was completely just but where justice was its only virtue would be a poor one and one not always to be preferred to other systems which had more and better books, less justly - perhaps even unjustly - distributed. For instance, too, it might be the case, say, that, in Northern Ireland, long term peace can be attained only by - contrary to justice - failing properly to punish some particular categories of criminals.

The Report is provocative rather than persuasive. It might serve as a stimulus for debate about public policies but not as an acceptable blueprint for the formulation and implementation of them. 'Social Justice' is a notion that functions for politicians and policy makers more agreeably as a source of vaguely defined 'visions' and as a rhetorical slogan rather than as a component part of specific arguments about particular competing policy recommendations.

I am tempted by the view that health and health related policy for Scotland should have a cluster of ends - the mains ones, I think, should be the treatment of illness and disease and the reduction of some sorts of pain and discomfort: the NHS should be, primarily, a National Sickness and Ill-health Service - and that the increase of the average life expectancy of the people of Scotland is not among them. If the effect of health policy is some increase (or reduction) in average life expectancy and/or the reduction (or increase) in health inequalities, then: so be it.

One of the aims of health policy should be to provide information relating to health regarding, for instance smoking, diet, exercise and drugs but this should be information on which people can choose to act or to fail to act rather than propaganda geared at the production of particular 'health gains' effects. The tone of the Green Paper is patronising and impertinent as, for instance, when it poses the question: 'How can smoking be stopped especially by young people and those living on low incomes who paradoxically smoke more and are least likely to stop.'[33] It is not the business of governments to 'combat smoking' nor to combat the legal elements of any chosen life style.

Notes

1.   *Working Together for a Healthier Scotland: A Consultation Document*, The Scottish Office Department of Health, (Edinburgh, 1998), The Stationery Office, Cm 3584, p.v.

2.   *Working Together for a Healthier Scotland: A Consultation Document*, p.vii.

3.   *Working Together for a Healthier Scotland: A Consultation Document*, pp.1-2.

4.   Susie Stewart (ed.), *The Possible Scot: Making Healthy Public Policy*, The Scottish Council Foundation, Paper No. 7 (1998).

5.   McLachlan, Hugh V., 'Justice, Rights and Health Care: A Discussion of the Report of the Commission on Social Justice', *International Journal of Sociology and Social Policy*, Vol. 18, Nos. 11/12, (1998).

6.   It was published under the title of Social Justice: Strategies for National Renewal It emanated from the Institute for Public Policy Research and was published in 1994. The members of the Commission and their occupations and/or affiliations as they were when the Commission sat were as follows:
Sir Gordon Borrie QC (Chairman of the Commission); Professor A.B. Atkinson FBA, Warden, Nuffield College, Oxford; Anita Bhalla, Asian Resource Centre, Birmingham; Professor John Gennard, Professor of Industrial Relations, Strathclyde University; The Very Reverend John Gladwin, Provost of Sheffield and Bishop-Elect of Guildford; Christopher Haskins, Chairman, Northern Foods Plc; Patricia Hewitt (Labour MP and a Secretary of the Treasury), Director of Research, Andersen Consulting; Dr. Penelope Leach, Fellow, British Psychological Society; Professor Ruth Lister, Professor of Social Policy and Administration, Loughborough University; Professor David Marquand, Professor of Politics and Director, Political Economy Research Centre, University of Sheffield; Bert Massie, Director, Royal Association for Disability and Rehabilitation; Emma MacLennan, Vice-Chairman, Low Pay Unit; Dr. Eithne McLaughlin, Reader in Social Policy, Queens University of Belfast; Steven Webb, Economist, Institute for Fiscal Studies; Margaret Wheeler, Director of Organisation Development, Unison; Professor Bernard Williams, FBA, White's Professor of Moral Philosophy, University of Oxford.

7.   Commission on Social Justice, *Social Justice: Strategies for National Renewal*, Vintage, (London, 1994), p.18.

8.   Commission on Social Justice, *Social Justice: Strategies for National Renewal*, Vintage, (London, 1994), p.18.

9.   Commission on Social Justice, *Social Justice: Strategies for National Renewal*, Vintage, (London, 1994), p.18.

10.   Commission on Social Justice, *Social Justice: Strategies for National Renewal*, Vintage, (London, 1994), p.18.

11.   Commission on Social Justice, *Social Justice: Strategies for National Renewal*, Vintage, (London, 1994), p.285.

12. Commission on Social Justice, *Social Justice: Strategies for National Renewal*, Vintage, (London, 1994), p.286.
13. Commission on Social Justice, *Social Justice: Strategies for National Renewal*, Vintage, (London, 1994), p.291.
14. Professor Le Grand is an adviser on health policy to the present Labour government.
15. See: McLachlan, Hugh V., 'Le Grand, Racism and the Nature of Equity', *International Journal of Sociology and Social Policy*, Vol. 15, No. 7.(1995).
16. McLachlan, Hugh V., 'The Right to Work', *Contemporary Review*, June, 1973.
17. Commission on Social Justice, *Social Justice: Strategies for National Renewal*, Vintage, (London, 1994), p.291.
18. Commission on Social Justice, *Social Justice: Strategies for National Renewal*, Vintage, (London, 1994), p.288.
19. Commission on Social Justice, *Social Justice: Strategies for National Renewal*, Vintage, (London, 1994), p.288.
20. Commission on Social Justice, *Social Justice: Strategies for National Renewal*, Vintage, (London, 1994), p.286.
21. Commission on Social Justice, *Social Justice: Strategies for National Renewal*, Vintage, (London, 1994), p.1.
22. Commission on Social Justice, *Social Justice: Strategies for National Renewal*, Vintage, (London, 1994), p.285.
23. Susie Stewart (ed.), *The Possible Scot: Making Healthy Public Policy*, The Scottish Council Foundation, Paper No. 7 (1998), p.4.
24. Susie Stewart (ed.), *The Possible Scot: Making Healthy Public Policy*, The Scottish Council Foundation, Paper No. 7 (1998), p.6.
25. *Working Together for a Healthier Scotland: A Consultation Document*, The Scottish Office Department of Health, (Edinburgh, 1998), The Stationery Office, Cm 3584, p.v.
26. *Working Together for a Healthier Scotland: A Consultation Document*, The Scottish Office Department of Health, (Edinburgh, 1998), The Stationery Office, Cm 3584, p.vii.
27. Commission on Social Justice, *Social Justice: Strategies for National Renewal*, Vintage, (London, 1994), pp.291-292.
28. Commission on Social Justice, *Social Justice: Strategies for National Renewal*, Vintage, (London, 1994), pp.288-289.
29. Susie Stewart (ed.), *The Possible Scot: Making Healthy Public Policy*, The Scottish Council Foundation, Paper No. 7 (1998), p.13.
30. Susie Stewart (ed.), *The Possible Scot: Making Healthy Public Policy*, The Scottish Council Foundation, Paper No. 7 (1998), p.12.
31. Susie Stewart (ed.), *The Possible Scot: Making Healthy Public Policy*, The Scottish Council Foundation, Paper No. 7 (1998), p.6.
32. Susie Stewart (ed.), *The Possible Scot: Making Healthy Public Policy*, The Scottish Council Foundation, Paper No. 7 (1998), p.6.
33. *Working Together for a Healthier Scotland: A Consultation Document*, The Scottish Office Department of Health, (Edinburgh, 1998), The Stationery Office, Cm 3584, p.vii, see also paragraph 121, and p.44.

8. The Provision of Healthcare in Remote Communities

JOHN CURNOW

In August 1930 the entire inhabitants of St Kilda abandoned their island home for a new and uncertain future on the mainland. What caused them to take such draconian steps was certainly complex. The process of decline in this close-knit community had begun many years before the Fishery Protection Vessel 'Harebell' and the steamer 'Dunara Castle' completed the evacuation on the 29th of August. By this time the population of the Island had fallen to less than forty individuals, many of who were elderly. The Islanders had always been poor and were dependent on two important factors for their survival. The first were the many seabirds colonising the dramatic cliffs around their home, which they slaughtered in their thousands for meat. The second was their benefactor, the Macleod of Macleod, who in exchange for a variety of Island produce provided seed and other essentials for life on St Kilda. The lifestyle here was so very different from almost any other part of the United Kingdom and it was not surprising that from time to time St Kilda was visited by curious folk anxious to capture the somewhat primitive scene. They brought with them welcome additional income for the community, but they were also responsible for more unfortunate consequences. The Islanders lacked immunity to infection and following such visits would often fall ill from the so-called 'boat-cold'. They had no doctor and illness was a serious matter here, even with the excellent attention of their resident nurse, Williamina Barclay.

Williamina, some years previous to the exodus, had predicted the fate of the Islanders, commenting that it was only a matter of time before they would all have to seek a safer existence. In the end it was probably the death of Mary Gillies from TB, a young lady in her twenties, which put the last nail in the lid of the Island's coffin. Atrocious weather had prevented her from being taken to the mainland for medical care. The death of one so young in the ageing community had a profound effect and a petition to the Government was raised requesting the resettlement of the entire population.

This document was entrusted for delivery to the care of the skipper of a passing trawler. Some months later the Islanders had their wish. To this day the Island remains without permanent inhabitants, apart from the seabirds that is, but fortunately it does have frequent visitors, some of them staying for extended periods.

Today the provision of healthcare in such a situation would be problematic and extremely expensive. However, surprisingly enough, many small populations throughout the United Kingdom are subject to conditions similar to those faced by the Islanders in 1930. In some ways the task of providing adequate access to the National Health Service for these people is even more difficult than arranging for medical attention then. Before we examine why this should be it is perhaps useful to consider just what we mean by a 'remote community'. It is surprising just how widely we can apply this definition throughout the United Kingdom.

Broadly, remoteness is a subjective quality but in National Health Service terms we can apply some operational stiffeners that should serve to move it towards a more objective stance. Geographical isolation is of course important but it is not the only consideration. Thus an offshore island set in calm waters with a good weather factor and a reliable means of transportation may not be considered as remote. Place the same Island at the same distance from the mainland in the North Sea and we have a very different situation. Poor weather in this case may significantly affect the ability to access more comprehensive medical services as frequently as is acceptable. Thus distance is only part of the over all equation. Transfer time to a clinical facility providing sufficient medical services is perhaps more useful.

Combine this with a weighting factor reflecting the difficulty in achieving transfer both in terms of cost and the ability to deliver the service throughout the year and we begin to define the problem. At this stage the nature and size of the population should also be considered. A risk assessment is required to assess the frequency with which such a transfer will need to be undertaken. Thus a small fit community at some considerable distance from the nearest hospital, for example a geological survey, will create less risk than a larger community reflecting the normal age distribution set much closer to the service. In the former case transfer is expensive, difficult but infrequent. In the latter situation the community will require NHS facilities at the usual population frequency and will need to travel more often. Prevailing conditions may very well prevent travel at certain times of the year and of course this applies to many mainland communities too. There are for example quite large mainland communities which because of prevailing conditions such as snow, or traffic congestion, occasionally become isolated for extended periods of time. The measure of a remote community therefore combines distance, or more properly transit time with a factor taking into account the difficulty in providing transport throughout the year coupled with the nature and size of the community.

How many such communities exist and why are they important? Actually these are difficult questions to answer. There are some very obvious examples of remote communities. One cannot fail to have noticed that the road from Tomintoul to Cock Bridge is frequently blocked by snow in the winter months. Other good examples can be found in Northern and Western Isles of Scotland, the Highlands and Grampian and in Wales and the West Country. These are the ones that come to mind readily but less straightforward are areas where specific local factors prevail to create isolation. For example, the residents of Newark on Trent on the Lincolnshire Nottinghamshire border have considered themselves isolated for some time because of the volume of traffic on the A1 Trunk road and adjacent routes, which effectively prevents them from getting to the University Hospital Nottingham in under an hour.

They are important because these communities often play a vital part in the local and national economy of the country as well as providing an alternative and arguably more satisfactory way of life, for families seeking different values from those associated with city life. They are also important because the Government says that they are. It has made its commitment to providing treatment for the people of Scotland 'where and when they want it' in the white paper *Designed to Care*. Whilst this is a laudable point of view any serious analysis of the problems of delivering medical services in such community will inevitably conclude that not all individuals can expect to receive all the care necessary for their well being in the immediate locality. Indeed under certain circumstances and for particular individuals a move closer to a specialist hospital is the sensible course of action. However, if too little medical provision is provided in the community many more of the population would begin to feel vulnerable and would follow the lead set by the St. Kilda Islanders in the 1930s. Getting the balance right is immensely important.

It is tempting to conclude that what is really required in these circumstances is a 'National Transfer Service' to provide an efficient means to transport patients from a distant community to a mainland hospital. There would appear to be obvious advantages in such a move. All that would be required remotely would be some system of triage in order to make a sensible decision as to which patient really required hospitalisation and which could be managed at home. A general practitioner or community nurse could easily achieve this and a good working arrangement with a large mainland hospital could provide all the secondary care needed for all but the most complex cases. In practice though, it is far more complicated.

To begin with, the local communities are almost always unhappy with this sort of arrangement. It effect on the ability of families to support a relative during a spell of sickness is one obvious and important factor. Also such an arrangement would involve the patient in several time consuming journeys to the hospital during the follow up phase of a hospital admission. Such a system would also be expensive to maintain. Sufficient travelling capacity would have to be arranged to cover both routine follow-up procedures and emergencies. Response times would have to be good enough to ensure that patients were not put at risk by unacceptable delays. If air travel were to be the mainstay sufficient pilot time would have to be available for a full 24-hour, 365 days a year, cover so the cost of providing for the emergency situation would be great. Inevitably, there would also be a proportion of inappropriate admissions. If the weather factor was poor the community would be effectively cut off from time to time and this would mean that some form of local arrangement would also have to be provided to cope when it was impossible to fly patients out. Escorting seriously ill patients and casualties is itself a skilled task requiring a good working knowledge of aviation and a feel for what is achievable in the air and what is not. Conditions in most aircraft used for aero-medical evacuation are such that there is little one can do for the patient once in the air. Some provision to ensure that patients were properly stabilised prior to take off would be absolutely essential. Putting all these things together we are led quite logically to the conclusion that at the very least there is a need for a facility that closely resembles a small community hospital, with enough trained staff to assess patients and stabilise them for transfer. They would also have to be able to cope safely with transfer delays. Anything less than this would almost certainly compromise patient safety. If such a unit were provided it would seem sensible to explore the possibility that it might also be used to provide limited secondary hospital care locally in addition to the emergency cover. Whilst this seems to a completely rational conclusion it raises other difficulties. Setting the level of local hospital activity is fraught with problems.

To illustrate the point it is useful to consider the situation in a real community. The Orkney Islands lend themselves readily to such an exercise since their geographical situation means they experience all the problems so far discussed. These islands are home to some twenty thousand people and are located, as any schoolchild will tell you, in a box at the top right hand corner of the map of the United Kingdom. They are subjected to some 'interesting' weather conditions; some pleasant but some far less so. The sea can sometimes be extremely rough.

Although most of the population is located on the main island or those islands linked by causeways, the Churchill Barriers, there is a significant minority living on a series of remoter Islands. These people travel to the main island by aeroplane or boat with journey times varying from twenty minutes to several hours. The islands have their very own local identity and population numbers are reasonably stable at this time. One important fact is that the internal island-to-island transport is not co-ordinated with the mainland air links. It should also be kept in mind that in the summer months the population of the islands is greatly increased by large numbers of visitors.

Health services are the responsibility of the Health Board, the smallest board in the United Kingdom, and it directly manages the diminutive and rather elderly hospital. The main stay of care in the community is the service provided by the GP's and their team. In addition the Local Authority provides essential facilities, for example community care for the elderly, in partnership with the Health Board. There are more general practitioners per head of population than on the Mainland. This is partly because of the small pockets of population on remote islands; a GP may only have a few hundred patients but he will be permanently on call. It is also because GP's are used in a slightly different way to their counterparts on the mainland. Practitioners in remote communities have to be more self-reliant and undertake a broader spectrum of duties, for example providing dispensing facilities. A high percentage of them are specially trained for trauma and emergency situations and they are expected to deal at the scene with accidents and acute medical emergencies. There is no doubt that these practitioners serve to stabilise the population by reassuring the community that health care will always be available. As we shall discover they are also finding themselves increasingly involved in managerial tasks as the structure of the particular form of island care evolves.

Orkney like so many other remote communities has, as previously described, a small hospital providing a basic range of medical and surgical services. In spite of the local facility transporting patients to mainland hospitals still accounts for some 5 per cent of the total healthcare budget. Determining the menu of locally available services is a fearsome task and has to take into account an assortment of issues surrounding professional pressures and patient safety. Nationally the trends are for greater numbers of specialised units providing, so the argument goes, centres of excellence with sufficient case throughput to ensure continued staff competence.

If we were to apply these principles strictly many Orkney patients would have to travel more frequently and even further afield for their treatment. The costs, in terms of both time and money would be considerable. Already for some patients a fifteen-minute outpatient appointment in Aberdeen means two days travelling with at least one overnight stop and for some the situation is even worse. The position would undoubtedly be improved if the internal travel timetables could be co-ordinated with flights connecting with the mainland. Even if this were achieved however, travel would remain a major consideration in service provision. Obviously bringing the mainland hospital team to the Island is an attractive alternative and indeed this is currently undertaken with some success. Naturally where sophisticated equipment and technology is required to assist diagnosis or treatment this may not be an option at this time. One must conclude that there is an ongoing need for remote hospital services and that they are likely to be fundamentally different to those being developed on the mainland. A more general approach is required embracing a number of disciplines vested in a small number of clinical staff.

The case for remote medicine as a specialty in its own right is indeed attractive. A medical colleague recently commented on his return from humanitarian duties in Central Africa that nothing he had experienced in medical school or during his training as a junior doctor had prepared him for what he had to undertake over there. The range of duties was staggering and the need was great. Equipment was limited and he frequently had to improvise. The demand on him far outstretched his experience. He was however able to transfer skills and, with a good reference book, carry out lifesaving procedures that he had rarely practised. Whilst one would not wish suggest that the circumstances in Orkney were anywhere near comparable with those in Central Africa, one cannot help wondering how much better prepared he would have been if he had spent some time here.

Perhaps one of the most difficult problems to overcome in a remote setting is that of professional isolation. This has a profound effect on the service and is a major aspect of the difficulties in recruiting medical and nursing staff to island posts. The perception of being out of the 'main stream' is a widely stated reason for not applying for such posts. More importantly the effect of distancing the individual from peers could lead to a drop in professional standards that would be totally unacceptable. To address these genuine concerns the use of modern technology in developing electronic links with major centres is of great potential benefit.

The use of such links in the educational process is going to become mandatory if remote centres are to continue to function. The operational benefits of providing a range of easily assessable experts to the remote clinician to assist in the management of patients are obvious. One of the exciting areas of tele-medicine is in the central interpretation of diagnostic procedures such as X-ray, ultrasound and ECG taken remotely. As well as making available the opinion of specialists to the Island physician such a system also serves to reduce the waiting time for such results. The support that this sort of technology provides clearly justifies a major investment. In the not too distant future we could see virtual ward rounds where the consultant staff, located in a major centre, participate fully in the management and clinical care of remotely situated patients.

Another inherent problem associated with island populations is that of scale. The cost of providing any medical service to such a community is high, measured by the conventional method of cost per head of population. In practice such communities are always disadvantaged because there is usually no minimum set up money linked to any development. Let us take an example. A creditable Scottish Executive initiative to reduce smoking related disease provides money for Health Boards to set up a service to encourage the population to give up cigarettes. Scotland has one of the worst records for smoking related disease in Europe and so this is an important initiative. Money is provided to the health board according to their population. For most Boards the funding is sufficient for the establishment of a specialist officer to manage the campaign with the appropriate support. For a small island board the money received is insufficient to even begin to address the task. Moreover if such a scheme required someone with specialist skill it is highly unlikely that such a person would exist locally, or could be attracted to a remote community on a part time basis. The community is thus doubly penalised.

Developing this important theme a little more it is clear that for any level of health care there will be a minimum staffing level necessary to meet the required provision. This would naturally include managerial and clinical skills for in this; island boards are no different to their larger mainland counterparts. But it is this that poses one of the greatest conundrums for often the small Boards simply cannot afford even the basic staff needed. We are then faced with the need to either employ staff on a part time basis or for individuals to assume more than one role. In practice this often results in a few people being responsible for many functions.

Funding for health boards in Scotland has historically been calculated using the SHARE Formula that sets out to redistribute money to boards on the basis of a set of needs-related criteria. However, increasingly the need-indices used are being questioned and it is apparent that due allowances for important factors such as remoteness and diseconomies of scale have not been incorporated. Recently the Arbuthnott Working Group reviewed the methodology employed in the resource allocation and some important changes have been recommended which go some way to rectifying the situation. However the smaller and remoter boards are still not properly provided for and it is perhaps questionable whether any single formula will meet the needs of health boards as diverse in size and character as Orkney and Glasgow.

It is also assumed that rural communities are significantly more fortunate, better off and healthier than their urban counterparts. Deprivation in general is considered to be a feature of cities and industrial complexes. Certainly rural deprivation is a completely different animal to urban deprivation but never the less just as potentially devastating to health and what is more it does exist. A family living in an isolated croft may not have electricity, a potable water supply, proper drainage or adequate heating, but the cottage would be classified as 'owner occupied'. The family might have to undertake several jobs to simply provide enough money to live. They might farm, fish, drive a taxi or school bus and provide emergency cover for a utility company. In statistical terms they are likely to be classified as self-employed owning their own property. In addition they are probably very reluctant to access the health service particularly if this might include a visit to the mainland hospital, with the prospect of a two-day journey. Such a trip would also take them away from their occupations so it is therefore not surprising that they are often reluctant to do this.

Of course this goes largely unrecognised, and only surfaces, at best, as an anecdotal tale. Sadly the public health function that should have recognised and properly recorded the anomaly is often in such areas so poorly developed as to be ineffectual. This again is a product of the Orkney Health Board not being able to afford what a bigger board would take for granted. We are therefore helping to perpetuate the myth that the rural population is a particularly healthy one.

At this point in time the reader may be forgiven if they conclude that the provision of health care in remote and rural populations is just too difficult and that the example shown by the residents of St Kilda in 1930 is by far the most sensible one. Perhaps it should be mandatory for everyone residing in the United Kingdom to live no more than five miles from a major teaching hospital.

Then again the reader may not necessarily appreciate the joys of driving to the office in the morning where the most taxing hazard has been a tractor and trailer. There are without a doubt some major hurdles to overcome if we are to retain adequate and acceptable levels of care in such communities. As we have discussed there are many factors working against such provision. The financial burden is high and the need for effective management is just as important in small remote areas as it is in more densely populated ones. The medical and nursing profession are moving for very laudable reasons towards specialisation and even super specialisation leaving the generalist as an endangered species. However, it is just such a being that remote and rural services are in need of.

Take for example the Island need for laboratory technology to support the hospital function. Almost everywhere else in the United Kingdom the hospital laboratory service is at the very least divided into clinical chemistry, haematology and microbiology with technicians specialising in one of these areas. On the Island our requirement is for someone who has a general competency in all three areas. Training and career patterns mean that it is very difficult to find such an individual. Of course there will also be an on going need to access the opinion of the relevant specialist in the larger hospital. The information technology necessary to assist small hospitals to supplement their diagnostic and treatment capabilities is available today and can be purchased 'off the shelf' so to speak. Frustratingly though at present there is little co-ordination or drive to capitalise on the benefits that such technology would bring.

The relationship between the small hospital in a remote and rural community and the larger provider hospital is an extremely important one but one that has suffered particularly badly as a consequence of the internal structure changes within the NHS. In the 'market place' health service there was little incentive to consider the particular needs of such communities and a mosaic of services was provided without proper consideration of real need. The situation was not helped by the lack of local statistics and needs related information and this inevitably lead to contracts and service agreements that were far from satisfactory. The net result was confusion and uncertainty on both sides leading to prickly dissatisfaction. If we are serious about providing medical support to these areas then this clearly cannot be allowed to continue.

Perhaps it is time to consider some solutions although it should be acknowledged from the outset that there is probably no single right answer. Again I will use the Orkney Islands as a focus but I would make it clear that the particular conditions prevailing here are probably quite different from other remote areas although the underlying principles are likely to be similar. Firstly the remote health care dilemma is probably too big to tinker around the edges and requires radical thought and novel solutions. This approach will impact upon the establishment and it is unlikely to do so quietly, but then conditions are rarely quiet for long in the Orkney Islands.

To deliver quality health care for an Island community we have to be very clear as to what can be managed locally, given the skills of the staff, the equipment and support available. This needs to be unambiguously recorded in protocols readily available to staff and agreed by colleagues in the mainland provider hospital. There may be occasions of course when circumstances conspire to prevent transfer of patients falling outside these protocols and so it is necessary to ensure that medical and nursing personnel receive training on a continuous basis to equip them for such events. How do you provide the necessary training for a general practitioner resident with his or her patients on a remote Island? The Islanders would regard any absence with some concern unless there was adequate locum cover. Again technology should be able to provide the answer. The development of Island seminars for medical and nursing staff based on video links overcomes the need for an unnecessary journey to the main island. Used regularly such a facility would help to overcome the professional isolation that a single-handed GP based on a small island might experience. There would also be the opportunity to discuss unusual cases, tapping into group expertise thus improving the clinical management of individual patients. The electronic network could easily extend to the mainland hospital expanding the teaching potential and ensuring that clinical results are received quickly.

We also have to be sure that when there is a need to access the mainland hospital in an emergency we have the means to do it. In practical terms this almost certainly involves the availability of an aircraft and crew for Orkney. In addition arrangements have to be in place to transfer from island to main island by fixed and rotary wing aircraft, or boat, as and when required.

In many parts of the world aero-medical evacuation has been used for years and is an essential part of sustaining communities in remote environments. In the United Kingdom opinion is divided as to the effectiveness of such a service with considerable attention being paid to its use in more densely populated areas. In Scotland it is indispensable. There are undoubtedly lessons to learn from other countries and the investment in the infrastructure here, both in terms of the hardware and the command and control has not been all that it could have been. Again the variable conditions under which air transport is being asked to perform really calls for a variety of aircraft types. Some of the airstrips in the Orkney Isles present challenging problems, particularly during the winter months when they may be waterlogged and obscured by low cloud. Even the scheduled passenger flights hold untold excitement when hopping between Islands at low level in poor visibility. Personnel used to escort patients require special training and although such training is available from a number of different sources there is no standardisation and the quality varies considerably. When faced with the evacuation of a large number of casualties the use of military aircraft, and their highly trained teams, would be an attractive option.

We are still faced with that most contentious of issues of providing primary and secondary care locally, which is both safe and affordable. Such care would have to be deliverable with the staffing levels and the skill mix available. It is here that a number of health service sacred cows need to be sacrificed. Essentially such provision is not achievable using a conventional approach with the current level of funding. Managers of the remote Health Service have but two options. Either they must plead for more revenue, or they must challenge the established mode of service delivery. The process of taking nothing for granted and expecting the medical and nursing profession to justify their stance with a whole lot of dogma, is not any easy one and is not likely to make many friends along the way. But fundamental questions do need to be asked. Why should we have primary and secondary care in the first instance when what we are really looking for is just 'Island care' which is seamless? Why shouldn't we use GPs to provide hospital medicine provided they have adequate support from a consultant physician? Can we ignore the fact that our surgeons need a wide repertoire of relatively minor procedures and that specialisation is actually counterproductive? Given the small population, is it really best use of resources to have two major agencies, the Health Board and the Local Authority, managing different components of care?

As a rule and most certainly in Orkney the Local Authorities and Health Boards do co-operate with each other in a highly effectual way and 'working together' is a stimulating experience, particularly in the provision of services for the elderly. Would it not, however, in the Island context, save valuable resources and be more efficient to have just one managing body? This remains an unanswered question at present. We have however begun to address the other issues. Recently we have embarked upon a new model of care in Orkney that does begin to breach the established barriers between primary and secondary care. The *Integrated Care Model* exploits the skills of the general practitioner and creates an environment for a whole range of additional activities within the hospital and in management. In choosing this route it is recognised that there will be a need to create support on an extensive scale and that much of this will have to come from mainland resources. Negotiations are underway with various bodies to win the much-needed professional recognition of the model. The programme of training is being developed to allow junior medical staff to take part in hospital activities as part of their general practice training. The comparatively recent formation of a *Remote and Rural Resource Centre* in Inverness opens up exciting possibilities and also establishes the opportunity to develop a focus for teaching and research.

In stating that remote and rural medicine is in someway different to mainstream medicine there is a need to ensure that it is both recognised by the establishment and adequately provided for. In particular training and accreditation require a major effort if we are going to encourage a fresh, high quality work force into this specialty. The partnership with larger hospitals has to be re visited and the needs of the remote and Island communities encapsulated within their mission statements. Ideally there should be a symbiotic relationship with the larger hospitals capitalising on the opportunities arising within their smaller partners. For even within major teaching hospitals there is a clear need for general experience. Even more fundamental is the need to ensure that medical students are exposed to the smaller hospital during their clinical years. Experience gained here would be invaluable and could form the basis of a wider understanding of community needs, possibly also going some way to equip individuals for such tasks as relief work in the future, should they require it. The importance of students and junior medical and nursing staff in rural hospitals cannot be overstated. Their challenge ensures that such hospitals grow in stature and understanding.

In looking at the wider issues of remote and rural medicine there are most certainly parallels with military medicine in that the skills required by the non specialist military doctor are just those needed in the Island environment. Recently the armed forces have suffered a medical manpower crisis with poor recruitment and retention being a serious feature. One of the proposed developments being considered by the military is the setting up of a College of Military Medicine. Since the two fields have considerable overlap it would be indeed tempting to consider some form of joint venture as the basis for continued expansion. As well as the obvious common features such as aero-medical evacuation, and the support of operations in remote theatres, the rather special skills associated with practising in the field while supported by an expert at a distance, could be developed.

No overview of a rural health service would be complete without considering the views of the population using the service. Quite rightly they want the best that the National Health Service can provide, and as conveniently positioned as is practicably possible. They are often surprised by the position taken by professional bodies and cannot entirely understand why this or that service cannot be provided locally, unless of course it is because it costs too much. The problem of continuing competence of medical staff faced with chronic lack of practice in managing rare conditions does not normally feature in their dialogue with the Board. The fact that a fully trained transplant team positioned in the hospital in Orkney today would be incapable of undertaking major surgery according to present guidelines in six months time is not widely appreciated; although I hasten to add that such a team would be able to deal with most ailments presenting for their attention. What are evident to them are the consequences of the decisions which the Board has to take in order to balance its budget. What is usually quite clear to the Board is the end result of having to decide between one course of action and another. Such shopping list decisions may pass unnoticed in a larger population but in the Islands they are usually visible in the extreme. Such banner headlines as 'Health Board taking God-like decisions' spring to mind. It is therefore absolutely essential that the island population be regarded as a working partner in what is an exciting journey into new health territory. That in itself is a challenge because in the great scheme of things it is comparatively easy to forget that the population is more than the inhabitants of the main island.

If we are to succeed in providing quality care for remote communities we are going to have to do a lot more than just leaving it to the local management to get on with it. There is no doubt that the cost of healthcare per head of population in such communities will be high. I believe it to be a worthwhile investment but only if it is properly supported at a national level. In Scotland with the benefit of the devolved parliament there is some appreciation of the value of such areas. Their important contribution to the economy of Scotland with regard to, farming, fishing, the Malt Whiskey industry and tourism is understood. Working with the Scottish Parliament to create a new model of care will undoubtedly be a challenge. The ability to co-ordinate elements described previously such as a national tele-medicine network will help to determine whether or not we will succeed in properly supporting these communities. Importantly it is the support that the larger hospitals are prepared to give which will be a major factor in the equation. It is indeed gratifying that at present there appears to be little of the malaise that befell the residents of St Kilda all those years ago evident in the population of the Orkney Islands.

9. Towards a History of the NHS in Glasgow and the West of Scotland: an Agenda for Future Research

MARGUERITE DUPREE

Charles Webster's definitive book on the early years of the National Health Service[1] gives a comprehensive overview of the advent of the NHS in terms of national policy formation and implementation, but the variations in experiences of the introduction of the NHS in different localities are only beginning to be explored systematically. These tend to focus on the regional hospital boards, the main administrative innovation of the new service and subject of reorganisation in 1974, and pay less attention to general practice and local authority provision.[2,3] The importance of a regional or local perspective is clear from John Pickstone's work, showing how local concerns and initiatives produced a distinctive, innovative pattern of development of psychiatric units in district general hospitals in Manchester around 1950, 'not in response to national policy but because of the way new *regional* decision-makers reacted to peculiar problems in the provision and staffing of mental health services.'[4] At the same time he stresses the importance of long-term patterns in the development of health services 'both generally and for features peculiar to the Manchester region'.

These two features provide a starting point for a future research project I am planning on the history of the NHS in Glasgow and the West of Scotland from 1948-1974. The principal aim of the research to examine in detail the changes the NHS brought in the administration of hospitals, general practice, local authority services, and medical education and how these changes were shaped and experienced in a particular location. This research will explore the ways in which the combination of the legacy of the long-term patterns of the provision of medical services, on the one hand, and the decisions of the new local and regional policy makers in the

138

face of particular problems on the other, shaped the provision of health care in a significant region, the Western Regional Hospital Board of Scotland centred on Glasgow. It will examine the changes and continuities in the administration of health services, in the range of services, in the experience of medical practitioners, medical students and patients after the 'appointed day' 5 July 1948 and up to the reorganisation in 1974. It will attempt to assess how big a transformation the advent of the NHS brought in the nature and mode of delivery of medical services.

The research will cover not only hospital services but also family practitioner services, local authority services and medical education. It is feasible because it focuses on a particular region, which can provide a microcosm for the examination of problems facing the new service and how they were met. Also, the research will not ignore patients, but it will concentrate on the medical community, particularly the medical practitioners. The legislation that created the NHS was perceived as a major upheaval in the provision of medical care; thereafter medical care was to be universal, comprehensive and free at the point of use. The study will examine how this medical community met these challenges. Finally, rather than regard the 'health-care system as a necessary by-product of developments in medical science' and technology as does much of the writing on the NHS,[5] the project provides an opportunity to examine the ways in which the health care system facilitated developments in medical science and shaped their translation into health care benefits.

Why Scotland and the West of Scotland?

Scotland is particularly suitable for such a study because there were significant differences between Scotland and England in the implementation of the NHS. First, there was separate legislation in Scotland which differed in several ways from that for England and Wales, notably the handling of hospital endowments (some of which were subsequently used to support research), and the placement of the ambulance services and of all hospitals, including the teaching hospitals, under Hospital Boards of Management and Regional Hospital Boards.[6] Arguably the integration of teaching hospitals with former local authority and voluntary hospitals facilitated the planning and management of specialist services and of medical innovations in Scotland, such as diagnostic ultrasound. The latter benefited from access to a wide range of patients in Glasgow hospitals and research funding from both the Scottish

Hospital Endowments Research Trust and the University of Glasgow.[7] It is also likely to have encouraged the regional development of postgraduate medical education.[8] Second, not only were there differences in legislation, but there were also differences in attitudes. Surveys reveal that practitioners in Scotland were more enthusiastic about both the 1911 National Insurance Act and the prospect of the NHS, than their colleagues in England.[9,10] The differential reaction of Scottish and English practitioners to the advent of the NHS continued after 1948, as few Scottish consultants were involved in private practice and hospitals did not encourage it, even though Bevan made allowance for private practice in the legislation. Currently, too, Scottish practitioners are less enthusiastic about recent changes, than those in England. Thus, the study provides an opportunity to examine the roots of major differences between Scotland and England.

At the same time that there were differences between Scotland and England, a study of the region covering the West of Scotland with Glasgow at its centre that came under the aegis of the Western Regional Hospital Board in 1948 offers features that make it representative not only of Scotland but also of other parts of the country. The region included approximately half of the population of Scotland and, with thirty-seven Hospital Boards of Management, was comparable in size with the larger English regional boards. Glasgow and the region surrounding it was also similar to the other Scottish regions surrounding Edinburgh, Aberdeen and Dundee where a striking feature was the large gap in population size and number of practitioners between the main city and the other towns in the region. One of the pre-conditions for the main part of the project is to examine the pre-existing regional basis of the organisation of medical care in the West of Scotland which the NHS institutionalised in 1948. Another reason to focus on Glasgow is the highly developed system of local authority hospitals and services existing on the eve of the NHS and its links with the University of Glasgow medical school. The University already used local authority hospitals for clinical teaching and the University department of Materia Medica and Therapeutics had been located in a local authority hospital since 1937. With the extensive development of local authority hospitals and services, it might be expected that the removal of hospitals from local authority control would be particularly difficult. In fact, as Alistair Tough mentions in his paper in this volume, the system of admission to former local authority hospitals remained centred on the 'Bar' at the headquarters of the Glasgow Public Health Department well into the 1950s, while the separate system of admission to former voluntary hospitals also continued primarily via referrals from general practitioners to consultants.[11] Also, contrary to accounts suggesting that those from the former voluntary hospitals dominated the new regional hospital boards, in Glasgow the first chairman of the Western Regional Hospital Board (1947-1955), Sir Alexander Macgregor, had been the Medical Officer of Health of Glasgow since 1925.[12] His prominence indicates that the voluntary hospitals might not have been dominant in Glasgow and suggests that it will be important to examine the backgrounds of the members of the new regional boards and hospital management committees. A further reason to focus on Glasgow is that like Edinburgh and London, it contained a major medical corporation, the Royal Faculty (from 1962 the Royal College) of Physicians and Surgeons of Glasgow. As the new history of the Royal College[13] describes, in Glasgow the University and College agreed on a division of labour with the former concentrating on undergraduate and the latter postgraduate medical education, offering specialist qualifications, increasingly important for those aspiring to consultant posts within the NHS.

The survival of sources further justifies the concentration of this study on Glasgow and the West of Scotland. The Greater Glasgow Health Board Archives (GGHB) are particularly rich, containing the minutes of the Western Regional Hospital Board and its committees and sub-committees; papers of the chairmen and secretaries; papers re: appointments to boards of management, annual reports, circulars, and news cuttings. Particularly valuable and unusual is the survival of the minutes and other papers of hospital boards of management. Also, surviving are the minutes, annual reports, press cuttings, etc. of the Executive Council for the City of Glasgow.

The Glasgow University Archives include the minutes and other papers of the Faculty of Medicine and the papers of Sir Hector Hetherington, Principal of Glasgow University who was Chairman of the Department of Health for Scotland's Committee on Post-War Hospital Problems in Scotland, 1942-1943 and a member of the Medical Education Committee for the Western Regional Hospital Area 1949-1950, including: papers and correspondence regarding the relationship between the University and the NHS; papers regrading University clinical appointments; correspondence and memoranda concerning the drafting of the NHS Bill for Scotland and the 'part the Universities ought to play in any organisation envisaged under the Bill'.

The Glasgow City Archives in the Mitchell Library hold the minutes of the Glasgow City Council and its committees, and some papers from the Public Health Department. The library and archives of the Royal College of Physicians and Surgeons of Glasgow, the Scottish Record Office in Edinburgh and Public Record Office at Kew also hold relevant papers. There is also a good collection of histories of individual hospitals and memoirs and autobiographies of contemporaries. Finally, the documentary sources also can be supplemented by interviews with key contemporaries.

Topics and Issues

This project will focus on Glasgow and the surrounding region in the West of Scotland under the control of the Western Regional Hospital Board during the period from 1948 to 1974. The main issues to be explored will be:

The Background

The regions under the NHS were deliberately centred on existing medical teaching centres and it will be an important preliminary background study for this project to illuminate the existing regional basis of the organisation of medical care in the West of Scotland. In order to do this within the time available, a preliminary study will focus on the interrelations between Glasgow's medical community and that of a typical town in its hinterland, such as Kilmarnock over approximately 80 years since 1870.

It is clear from previous work using the 1911 Medical Directory[14] that registered medical practitioners were concentrated in the four major Scottish cities, and one of the striking features of regions surrounding these cities is the large gap in population size and number of medical practitioners between the major city and the other towns in the region. For example in the West of Scotland Glasgow had a population of 564,968 in 1891, and while Kilmarnock had a population of 28,438 in 1891 or about 5 per cent of the Glasgow population. This part of the project will use the methodology of Hilary Marland's excellent comparative study of medical communities[15] in which she compares medical services in two medium-size Yorkshire towns with different economic and social structures. Her study, however, leaves in the shadows these towns' place in the regional hierarchy of medical practitioners and institutions centred on Leeds, so her method will be adapted to examine the extent of Glasgow's regional influence and the ways it operated, as well as used to compare the two different medical communities. It is likely that there was a regional organisation and delivery of medical services, with for example, citizens in Kilmarnock subscribing to Glasgow voluntary hospitals and the medical practitioners in Kilmarnock and similar towns tending to be trained in Glasgow, referring patients to Glasgow hospitals, joining Glasgow-based medical societies or inviting Glasgow-based speakers to local medical societies. A hypothesis to explore is that these links in turn may have led to regional styles of medical treatment and care.

The Coming of the NHS

Having explored the regional background of the NHS, the project will examine changes in the three main sectors of the NHS - the hospitals, the local authority services, and the general practitioner services - as well as in medical education.

Hospitals

The main issues to explore with regard to the hospitals include:
(a) Changes in the administrative structure - The changes in the administrative structure of hospitals were the major administrative innovation of the NHS legislation. What changes did the new structure bring to Glasgow and the West of Scotland? Which hospitals were included and which (for example, private nursing homes) were excluded from the control of the Regional Hospital Board? How were hospitals grouped into Hospital Boards of Management? What were the WRHB's relationships with central government on the one hand and with Hospital Boards of Management on the other?
(b) Appointment and Membership of Western Regional Hospital Board (WRHB) and Hospital Management Committees - How were the members of these boards appointed? What were the members' backgrounds (occupation, place of residence, medico-political, political)? To what extent did they represent voluntary hospital interests? How frequent was the turnover of members?
(c) Medical Practitioners - How were consultants appointed in all hospitals? Who were appointed consultants - previous staff of hospitals, general practitioners? Did they give up private practice? To

what extent were general practitioners in Glasgow and the West of Scotland excluded from hospitals? Within local authority hospitals how was the change in the structure from the medical superintendent controlling salaried medical staff to the new structure based on consultants implemented?

(d) Specialist Units - To what extent was the model of the general hospital with specialist units implemented, particularly in specialities such as orthopaedics which Roger Cooter has shown had non-hospital treatment, such as rehabilitation, as part of the concept of the speciality before the NHS?[16] To what extent were specialist units developed to serve the entire region, for example plastic surgery at Cannisburn Hospital?

(e) Admissions:

(i)   How were patients admitted to hospitals? To what extent did pre-1948 patterns continue, such as: the 'Bar' (the system for admitting patients to local authority general hospitals after these hospitals were removed from the Poor Law in the 1930s as mentioned above); referral (facilitated by informal contacts, such as general practitioners and consultants playing golf together); and the exclusion of certain types of cases, such as the elderly, from general hospitals? To what extent did the arrangements change, for example, from the rotating allocation of emergency beds among voluntary hospitals to all beds allocated so there was no room for emergency cases?[17]

(ii) To what extent and for what conditions did demand for hospital beds increase? How was this met? There is evidence that the 'acute' general hospitals excluded patients over age 65; this helped stimulate alternative facilities and geriatric medicine. Also, how long did the local authority 'Bar', subject to influence from local councillors, continue for admitting patients to former local authority hospitals?[18] In short, how was the 'locus of caring' determined?

(f) Regional Services such as the Department of Clinical Physics will be examined.

(g) Voluntary work within hospitals - The Glasgow Hospitals Auxiliary Association was established in 1948 to continue the tradition of voluntary work within the NHS. What services did it provide and how did they compare with those before the NHS?

(h) Other issues will be investigated if time allows, for example: Did the NHS bring an increase and redistribution of capital and equipment expenditure among hospitals? What role did the WRHB play in the formation of the 'Hospital Plan for Scotland' of 1962 and what effects did it have? To what extent did the roles and conditions of nurses and other staff change?

Local Authority

Many questions arise regarding local authorities including:
(a) To what extent were previous local authority services for particular groups, such as the mentally deficient and the elderly, reduced and eliminated by the NHS? In Glasgow from 1931 the local authority provided an outdoor medical service with clinics for the elderly which were eliminated under the NHS when medical services were transferred to the WRHB.[19]
(b) How easily were the new boundaries between the local authority services and the hospital and the family practitioner services implemented? There were problems, for example, with the distinction between the 'sick' and 'infirm' elderly, which divided responsibilities; also those who were classified as 'frail but ambulant' were not well catered for.[20]

General Practice

The experience of general practitioners, too, raises many questions:
(a) The prospect of the NHS: What was the attitude of general practitioners in Glasgow and the West of Scotland to the prospect of the NHS? How divided was opinion? What were their hopes and fears? Were general practitioners in Glasgow as anxious as one in London who experienced symptoms of duodenal ulcer for the first time in his life in the months leading up to July 1948 which disappeared shortly afterwards never to recur?[21]
(b) What difference, if any did the end of the sale of practices make to finding a practice? Did Executive Councils in the West of Scotland carry over membership and procedures from the National Insurance system, as has been suggested in the general literature?
(c) To what extent and from what groups did demand for the services of general practitioners increase? How was the demand met?

(d) To what extent were practices in Glasgow and the West of Scotland single-handed? What was their geographical distribution? Did the NHS lead to an increase in group practices?

(e) Did general practitioners in the West of Scotland have hospital appointments, for example as anaesthetists, that they had to relinquish with the coming of the NHS? Were they cut off from hospital services, such as diagnostic services, which they previously utilised?

Medical Education

Issues surrounding medical education to explore include:

(a) What effect did the NHS have on the existing University departments and personnel and arrangements for clinical teaching of undergraduates? What role did Sir Hector Hetherington, the Principal of Glasgow University play? He was a central figure in shaping medical education and its relationship to the hospitals. He was Chairman of the Department of Health for Scotland's Committee on Post-War Hospital Problems in Scotland, 1942-1943, gave evidence to the Goodenough Committee on Medical Education (1944 encouraged the Department of Health in Scotland to implement recommendations of the Goodenough Committee not to fund the extra-mural medical schools in Glasgow which led to their closure and the elimination of their students from competition for clinical teaching, relieving, for example, shortage of maternity beds. He also served on the Medical Education Committee of the Regional Hospital Board in its early years.

(b) In what ways did the NHS influence the development of postgraduate medical education, by, for example, including the teaching hospitals in the WRHB or by setting up central services for the region such as that for clinical physics which set up training courses for the use of ultrasound? What relationships developed between the WRHB, Glasgow University and the Royal College of Physicians and Surgeons of Glasgow?

(c) Professor Ferguson Anderson organised geriatric medicine within the WRHB and held the first chair of geriatric medicine in the world established in 1965 at Glasgow University. Recent scholarship has identified the previously unrecognised importance of Professor Anderson and other geriatricians in Scotland in the history of geriatric medicine in the UK and world-wide. The work of these geriatricians, for example, on the nature of the normal ageing process as well as the diseases of old age was highly significant. What institutional structures peculiar to Scotland and Glasgow in particular facilitated or hindered this research and associated innovations in the organisation of care?

Chronological, Regional and Analytical Limitations

The full potential of this regional case study, however, will only be realised if the local research is allied to a broad concept of health care and its evolution both at a national level and throughout the period as a whole.

Chronological

It will try to avoid too great an emphasis on the background and the setting up of the NHS and give due consideration to the1960s when a generational change in the medical profession and an increase in resources made an attack on its historical legacy possible.

Regional

There is a danger that the minutiae of administrative developments and battles (however important some may be symbolically) may obscure the broader political economy in which policy was framed, particularly in the 1960s. Then a greater emphasis on planning, particularly the work of the Public Expenditure Survey Committee, made explicit the range of options and priorities being addressed and determined - including disagreements between the Scottish Department of Health and the Ministry of Health on the balance between hospital and local authority services. More generally it is important to put Glasgow and the West of Scotland into the context of how the NHS in Scotland was run and the role of the Scottish Office and whether the BMA in Scotland had views which differed from those of its headquarters in London. Local studies need to reflect the changing national UK and Scottish picture and require adequate research in national as well as local archives.

Analytical

The emphasis of the project outlined above is on politics and administrative structures and the producers of health care, rather than on the outcome of policy. This will need to be modified and the provision of medical care will also need to include the evolving relationship between the NHS and social work and the extent of medical advice on, and intervention in, broader issues such as housing and pollution, with their major influence on health outcome.

By the time the NHS reaches its next significant anniversary there should be far more known about the regional variations in its implementation, development and consequences, and the extent to which these were shaped by the Scottish Office in Edinburgh and local and national politics. We also should know more about the inter-relationships among the hospital services, family practitioner services, local authority services and medical education.

Notes

1. Webster, Charles, *The Health Services Since the War*, (London, 1988).
2. Brown, R. G. S. *Reorganising the National Health Service: a Case Study in Administrative Change*, (Oxford, 1979).
3. Ham, Christopher *Policy-Making in the National Health Service: a Case Study of the Leeds Regional Hospital Board*, (London, 1981).
4. Pickstone, John, 'Psychiatry in District General Hospitals: History, Contingency and Local Innovation in the Early Years of the National Health Service' in John Pickstone (ed*), Medical Innovations in Historical Perspective*, (Basingstoke and London, 1992), pp.185-199.
5. Webster, Charles 'Conflict and Consensus: Explaining the British Health Service', *Twentieth-Century British History* 1 (1990), pp.132-133.
6. Webster, Charles, *The Health Services Since the War*, (London, 1988), p.104.
7. Dow, D. A. and John Lenihan,, 'The Impact of Technology' in McLachlan, Gordon (ed), *Improving the Common Weal: Aspects of Scottish Health Services 1900-1984*, Edinburgh, 1987) pp.505-528.
8. Stevens, R. *Medical Practice in Modern England: the Impact of Sp[ecialisation and Stat Medicine*, (New Haven and London, 1966), p.169.
9. Jenkinson, J., M. *Medical Societies in Scotland*, (Edinburgh, 1992), pp.99-103.
10. Hamilton, D. N. H. *The Healers: A History of medicine in Scotland*, (Edinburgh, 1987), pp.260-261.
11. Watt, Oliver, *Stobhill Hospital: the First Seventy Years*, Glasgow, 1971, WRHB Minutes, 2 June 1948.
12. Macgregor, Alexander *Public Health in Glasgow 1905-1946*, (Edinburgh, 1967).
13. Hull, A., and J. Geyer-Kordesch, *The History of the Royal College of Physicians and Surgeons of Glasgow 1858-1999*, (Glasgow, 1999).
14. Dupree, M. W. and A. Crowther, 'A Profile of the Medical Profession in Scotland in the Early Twentieth Century: the *"Medical Directory"* as a Historical Source', *Bulletin of the History of Medicine* 65 (1991), pp. 209-233.
15. Marland, Hilary, *Medicine and Society in Wakefield and Huddersfield 1780-1870*, (Cambridge, 1987).

16. Cooter, R., *Surgery and Society in Peace and War: Orthopaedics and the Organization of Modern Medicine 1880-1948*, (Basingstoke and London, 1993).

17. GGHB HB28/15/2, 'The Chronic Sick in Hospital', March 1954.

18. Watt, Oliver, *Stobhill Hospital: the First Seventy Years,* (Glasgow, 1971).

19. Anderson, Ferguson 'Geriatrics' in McLachlan, Gordon (ed), *Improving the Common Weal: Aspects of Scottish Health Services 1900-1984,* (Edinburgh, 1987), pp. 367-381.

20. McLachlan, Gordon (ed), *Improving the Common Weal: Aspects of Scottish Health Services 1900-1984,* (Edinburgh, 1987), pp. 367-381.

21. Hale, Geoffrey and Nesta Roberts, *A Doctor in Practice,* (London and Boston, 1974), pp.125,127.

10. The first 50 years of the NHS in Scotland. A less celebratory view

ALISTAIR TOUGH

During its anniversary year, much was written about the first 50 years of the National Health Service. By and large the tone has been celebratory, even congratulatory. That this should have been the case is unsurprising. It is particularly unremarkable in Scotland where the NHS continues to serve the vast bulk of the population. In contrast to the situation in the South of England where the NHS increasingly provides emergency services and services for the socially marginalised – the elderly, the impoverished and the chronically sick – the NHS in Scotland is still relied upon by the majority of successful middle class families. In this it represents an enduring memorial to British wartime social solidarity and cross-party consensus. After all, the NHS was a war baby. Its creation was recommended by Sir William Beveridge, a Liberal, in his famous report on social services published in 1942. This was accepted by the Conservative led wartime coalition and implemented by Nye Bevan - Health Minister in the post-war Labour Government.

I hope here to provide a less celebratory, and therefore more balanced, summary account of the achievements and weaknesses of the NHS in Scotland, and especially in Glasgow and the West of Scotland.

When the NHS was launched in 1948 a huge reservoir of sickness and distress was revealed. Doctors' surgeries overflowed with patients who had long-standing problems - women with prolapsed uteruses, men with huge hernias, nearly deaf people who had no hearing aids. Dentists faced a tidal wave of people who had bought ill-fitting second hand dentures in junk shops and at jumble sales. Meanwhile, opticians struggled to cope with those who wore second hand spectacles and had never had an eye test. The cost of dealing with this accumulated backlog of illness was great.

Beveridge had estimated that the new NHS would cost £150 million a year for Britain as a whole. The Government had set aside £200 million. In reality the NHS cost £450 million in its first full year of operation. The NHS has operated under severe budgetary constraints ever since. This has been particularly true of the capital budget and this in turn has served to make conflicts between particular parts of the NHS acute.

In 1948 there was general optimism about the future. Although there was food rationing and a chronic housing shortage and bomb damage was visible almost everywhere, there was also full employment, wage levels were high and British exports were in demand throughout the world. Crucially, people felt that the old fears of hunger, poverty and sickness had been lifted by the new welfare state. At an early stage, however, doctors became concerned that patients were becoming 'medicine-mad'. So extreme were the demands from some patients that the Department of Health for Scotland printed posters for the doctors' surgeries, which said "The Health Service cannot provide you with household remedies. If you wish to keep a store of such things as cotton wool, bandages, aspirins and laxatives at home, you must buy them yourself."

It would be wrong to say that only wealthy people could afford to be sick before the NHS was created. Most working men were covered by a National Health Insurance scheme introduced by the Liberal Government before 1914. Many women and children were cared for by works schemes such as the Lanarkshire Collieries Medical Services Association or by 'club' doctors - under cheap private insurance clubs. Some councils had particularly good services, for example Glasgow Corporation provided elderly people with a comprehensive service of home helps, district nurses and salaried doctors. In other words, before 1948 provision was very patchy. Many people, especially women, children and elderly people were not entitled to free treatment and could not afford doctors' fees. Many more did not understand what they were entitled to and stayed away out of ignorance and fear. The creation of a national service was intended to sweep away these fears.

The NHS brought sweeping change for doctors too. The most eminent doctors had previously relied on private patients for their income. Their hospital jobs were honorary and they usually only spent 3 hours a day with hospital patients. The rest of their time was devoted to paying patients. In Glasgow these 'consulting physicians' and 'consulting surgeons' usually lived near Charing Cross. It was to surgeries within their homes that the paying patients came for consultations. In Edinburgh and Aberdeen too the top members of the profession worked from fashionable West End addresses. Even Professors of Medicine were mostly part timers before

1948. They spent 3 or 4 hours a day on teaching students and attending to patients in the university teaching hospitals. The rest of their time was devoted to paying patients. The NHS simultaneously reduced the number of patients willing to pay and created full-time jobs for consultants. The result was a rapid expansion of medical and surgical specialisms. Plastic surgery, brain surgery, urology, dermatology and many other specialisms flourished as never before. The NHS, working with the universities, funded regional specialist centres like Canniesburn Hospital where major advances in plastic surgery were pioneered and doctors from across the Commonwealth came to study.

Medical imaging is one specialised area in which Scotland has made a particular contribution to worldwide medical and scientific advance. Ultrasound, which makes it possible for parents to "see" their unborn child, was pioneered in Glasgow during the 1950s by a multi-national and multi-skilled team led by Professor Ian Donald, a South African. His helpers included a doctor, an engineer and a clinical physicist. NMR (Nuclear Magnetic Resonance) imaging was developed in Aberdeen during the 1970s by a team led by Professor John Mallard who first demonstrated the equipment in action in 1980.

In the 1950s there was a belief that the NHS would put itself out of business. Advances in medical science coupled with better housing and nutrition were expected to create a much healthier population. So far as infectious diseases are concerned this actually did happen. Tuberculosis was virtually eliminated by a combination of new drug treatments and mass X-ray screening. Poliomyelitis, diphtheria, whooping cough, scarlet fever and measles - all of which had once struck terror into the hearts of parents - were similarly defeated during the first two decades of the NHS.

On the basis that a healthier population would need fewer hospitals, Governments were reluctant to provide the infant NHS with an adequate capital budget. The inevitable result was severe conflict over the use of money. In this fight the university teaching hospitals and regional specialist centres generally came out on top. The losers were the geriatric and psychiatric hospitals. Standards of hospital-based geriatric care had generally been low before 1948. Even in the late 1950s many still functioned like Victorian poor law institutions. Particularly discouraging both for staff and patients was the widespread perception that people went there to die: that there could be no question of treating and discharging their patients. In this context, the loss of Glasgow's domiciliary medical service for the elderly was particularly tragic. The service had been created in the early 1930s, using permissive powers in the 1929 Local Government (Scotland) Act. Salaried doctors, nurses and support staff provided what would later be termed 'care in the community'. Initially the patients included many unemployed people and their families but as unemployment levels dropped the service became de facto a domiciliary medical service for the elderly. When the NHS was created in 1948, the Glasgow service had to be dismantled because the British Medical Association had a fixed objection to salaried service. They had struck a national deal under which family doctors would be independent contractors. Sir Alexander McGregor, first Chairman of the regional hospital board and previously Medical Officer of Health for Glasgow, understood the calamity which this represented but could find no way of avoiding it under the cumbersome bureaucratic structures of the NHS.

In psychiatric hospitals the problems were particularly acute because of inadequate nursing staff levels. Ironically these were partly the result of improvements in staff working hours. In wartime, hospital nurses' hours had been reduced to 48 hours per week. To make up for this, additional staff were urgently needed. They could not be recruited because there was a chronic shortage of accommodation in the nurses' homes and it was virtually impossible for the nurses to live out because the psychiatric hospitals were located in such remote places. This was the direct consequence of two causes. Firstly, the provision of an inadequate capital budget for the NHS. And, secondly, the success of the teaching hospitals and specialist centres in monopolising what little capital was available. In the 1950s it was not unknown for a single nurse to be left in charge of 50 patients with severe learning difficulties for an entire eight-hour shift, with little prospect of support or relief from either nursing or medical colleagues. Naturally, the quality of service that could be provided was not high. Eventually the crisis in the psychiatric hospitals was eased by advances in drug therapy. As anti-depressant, anti-psychotic and mood-stabilising drugs became available so care in the community became a viable alternative to institutionalisation.

During the 1960s a growing crisis amongst general practitioners led to demands for a thorough reorganisation of the NHS. When the health service was first set up the hospitals had become the responsibility of one NHS administration while family doctors, dentists, opticians and pharmacists had been made the responsibility of a separate sector. District nurses, the schools health service and public health matters had remained with local councils. The weaknesses of this division of administration between 3 sectors had been shown by the very slow progress achieved in the creation of health centres. The local councils were supposed to take the lead in constructing health centres, which would house family doctors, district nurses, health visitors and dispensing chemists. Some progress was made - at Sighthill in Edinburgh and in Stranraer, for example - but many councils demonstrated a marked lack of enthusiasm which verged on obstructionism. The Medical Officers of Health, having seen their hospitals nationalised by the NHS, were not at all keen to build health centres, which they suspected would be confiscated in a similar manner. As slum clearance progressed and peripheral housing estates proliferated in the 1960s, so the failure to create health centres to cater for the new residential areas became a matter of acute concern. The end result was a comprehensive reorganisation in the mid 1970s which produced an integrated NHS administration.

Since 1974 reorganisation has become a persistent feature of life in the NHS. Districts have come and gone. Units have been created, amalgamated and abolished. General management has been introduced, NHS Trusts have been created and an internal market has been created and then, seemingly, abandoned. Sometimes it seems to those who work in the health service that they operate in an environment of perpetual revolution.

In the mid 1950s the rising cost of funding the NHS prompted the Government to appoint a committee to look for ways of cutting expenditure. When Professor Guillebaud and his committee reported they shocked ministers by saying that the NHS, whilst imperfect, represented very good value for money. Their influential report recommended an increase in the budget, not least for new hospitals. The consequent 'Hospital plan for Scotland' was launched by a Conservative Government in the late 1950s and embraced by the incoming Wilson Government in 1964. Under the plan, District General Hospitals were to be built in most major towns. Over the following years many new hospitals like Monklands General in Coatbridge and the re-built Royal Alexandra Infirmary in Paisley were opened. These had a profound significance for the large infirmaries in the main cities. Many patients who would previously have been treated in Aberdeen, Dundee, Glasgow or Edinburgh were now being taken into hospitals nearer to their homes. Only those with particularly severe injuries or complicated or rare illnesses are now sent from outlying areas to the big teaching hospitals like Ninewells in Dundee, Forresterhill in Aberdeen or the Southern General in Glasgow. A policy of revenue equalisation has accompanied the redistribution of the workload away from the large city hospitals. In Glasgow especially the movement of population out of the metropolis to satellite towns has further accentuated the redistribution of resources.

International comparisons show that the NHS offers good value for money. In the USA people spend on average 14 per cent of their income on health care. In Britain the figure is 7 per cent. Yet life expectancy is slightly higher in Britain whilst infant mortality is lower. Despite this, the NHS is constantly the subject of criticisms and complaints and always has been. Aneurin Bevan, the Health Minister who launched the service foresaw this. He said:

'We shall never have all we need. Expectations will always exceed capacity. [The NHS] ... must always be changing, growing and improving: it must always appear inadequate.'

Looking back over the first 50 years of the NHS, it seems to me that accountability is an outstanding challenge to the Service. Prior to 1948, local authority health services were scrutinised by elected councillors and the staff of the voluntary hospitals was accountable to those who supported them with their subscriptions. Since 1948 no really effective mechanism of accountability has been devised. In my opinion those appointed to serve on the various boards of management and so on have suffered both from being part-timers and from being appointed rather than elected. The weakness of the formal management structures has created a power vacuum and the service providers, particularly the leaders of the medical profession, have filled it. I have attempted to describe how the low standards of care in geriatric medicine and psychiatry, which prevailed in the past, were due, in part, to the excessive influence of leading specialists. It would be unfair, however, to place excessive blame on the latter. They were only seeking what they believed to be best for their patients. The negative consequences flowed from weak management and an inadequate level of accountability to the public as a whole. Rectifying this situation is one of the most important challenges facing the recently created Scottish Parliament.

Notes

This article is not the product of a preconceived research design nor of an a priori analytical framework. Rather it is the result of eight years spent looking after the archives of hospitals, clinics and NHS administrations in the Greater Glasgow area. I have been influenced by many conversations with doctors, nurses and other members of staff of the NHS, both current and retired, by a wide range of publications, by contemporary political debate, by participation in seminars and conferences, by the questions posed by users of the Greater Glasgow Health Board Archives (especially students and research fellows of the Wellcome Unit for the History of Medicine in the University of Glasgow). I am much indebted to all of those who have stimulated my thinking but none of them bear any responsibility for my conclusions.

11. Beveridge in Holland. National, Corporatist and Market Forces in Dutch Health Care

GEERT DE VRIES, MAARTEN VAN BOTTENBURG AND
ANNET MOOIJ

For all we know, Sir William Beveridge never visited Holland. He did to some extent, though, influence the course of the development of the Dutch welfare state. The famous blueprint Social Insurance and Allied Services in 1942 not only impressed the British people but also the Dutch government, which had fled the German Occupation and resided in London at the time. Still in exile, it installed its own Commission, chaired by the Secretary General of the Ministry of Social Affairs, Dr. A.A. van Rhijn. Inspired by the Beveridge report, the Van Rhijn Commission produced a preliminary proposal for a comprehensive post-war social security system in The Netherlands. The proposal was published in Holland soon after the Liberation. Hopes were high for fundamental changes in Dutch society. Soon, however, pre-war political powers reaffirmed their grip. As a consequence, the post-war system of social security in The Netherlands turned out to be much more an extension on pre-war foundations than a radical break, like the National Health Service in the United Kingdom. Nonetheless, the Dutch post-war system of social security was influenced by the war. Somewhat to our collective embarrassment, the Germans put a deeper stamp on it than the British did. This goes especially for the domain of social health insurance. We will present a brief overview of its development in The Netherlands over the past fifty years. We hope that the differences and the similarities between the United Kingdom and The Netherlands will stimulate further discussion.

The situation before the German Occupation[1]

In the nineteenth century and the beginning of the twentieth, a great variety of 'ziekenfondsen' or sickness funds existed in The Netherlands. They provided a very limited insurance against the costs of illness for the working classes - but not for those on the lowest incomes, who could not afford even a small insurance premium. Private insurance companies provided broader insurance schemes for those on higher incomes.

By the 1920s and 1930s, this variety of funds had crystallised into three main categories:
(1) 'maatschappijfondsen', i.e. funds collectively under the control of the (Royal) Dutch College of Physicians (K)NMG[2] and each one individually governed by a majority of doctors;
(2) 'onderlinge' or mutual funds governed by those insured themselves and loosely affiliated to the socialist and the protestant trade unions;
(3) Roman Catholic funds governed by Roman Catholic trade unions and indirectly by the RC church.[3]

Historically, the 'maatschappijfondsen' and the 'onderlinge' had been the first to organise themselves in reciprocal animosity, each fearing the other's growing influence. Then, for fear of lagging behind, the Roman Catholics had followed suit, thus completing a configuration of triangular rivalry.[4]

Two different antagonisms divided the parties. On the one hand there was the class struggle between doctors and the funds dominated by them (the Dutch Medical Society NMG with its 'maatschappijfondsen') and those insured (the workers) and their funds (both the mutual funds and the catholic ones) on the other. At he same time there was the religious competition between non-catholics (the NMG, the 'maatschappijfondsen' and the mutual funds) on one side with the catholics (the Roman Catholic funds) on the other.

The 'maatschappijfondsen' were the largest in number. Together with the Dutch Medical Society - or rather the other way around: the Medical Society, together with the funds it controlled - and they could often enforce their will across the field of social sickness insurance. Similarly, they could nearly always block radical proposals from the other parties, such as proposals for universal insurance schemes, for having doctors work as employees of sickness funds or in state employment, or for the free catchment areas that catholic funds were always wanting. Sickness funds had always had strong local roots. Even when they grew in size, they tended to stick to their original catchment areas: mergers occurred within these areas, not between them. Only the Catholic funds, concentrated in the south of The Netherlands, strove towards expansion, in order to rescue catholic workers' souls in the north from the corrupting influences of protestant or neutral funds. The fact that in the field of Dutch health insurance and health politics in general, doctors enjoyed double representation: directly through their own Dutch Medical Society, and indirectly via the 'maatschappijfondsen' that were more or less owned by them, was of cardinal importance.

The political arena was no less complicated than the world of the sickness funds. From the inception of universal suffrage - women were allowed to vote in 1919 - with the system of proportional representation, no single political party in The Netherlands has ever attained an absolute majority. Coalition governments have ruled throughout the twentieth century. Up until 1938 coalitions consisted of liberal-conservative, protestant and/or roman catholic political parties. After 1938 and especially after 1945 the Social Democratic party became a serious player as well. In fact the slow growth of the Dutch welfare state before the Second World War has been attributed to the ruling of the afore-mentioned liberal-conservative confessional governments, while its rapid expansion after the War has been attributed to the fact that the social democrats began to take part in coalitions. This does not mean that the social democrats alone were responsible for the expansion, but rather that their sheer presence as coalition candidates forced the other parties, especially the confessional ones, into vote competition. The Dutch welfare state is of mixed descent and has much christian democrat blood in its veins. In the 1960s even the liberal-conservatives were drawn into this competition: they could no longer afford to oppose generous welfare arrangements. Of course, within ten years the game of credit claiming would change into an altogether different game of blame avoidance.[5]

But let us return to the situation before the War. While several governments and individual ministers had tried to impose order upon the heterogeneous field of collective health insurance, and while many initiatives had been taken by players within this field (notably by the NMG, the mutual funds and trade unions), nothing had been achieved. Doctors fought any infringement upon their individual and professional autonomy and resisted attempts to raise the income limits for membership of sickness fund insurance, in order of course to safeguard the profitability of their private practices. Sickness funds solicitated state regulation and subsidies on the one hand, but feared state interference on the other. Their ideal was a typically Dutch one: to be the master of your own house, while charging the state for the costs of it.[6] This fortunate state of affairs had been achieved in the field of education, where besides state schools, protestant and roman-catholic schools had become fully subsidized while retaining their autonomy. In the field of sickness insurance, the state carefully refrained from burdening itself with financial obligations.

The Sickness Fund Decree of 1941[7]

Much to the discomfort of post-war generations, the first national scheme of collective health insurance in The Netherlands was introduced by the Germans who occupied the country from May 1940 until May 1945. In 1941 they proclaimed the so-called 'Ziekenfondsenbesluit' (Sickness Funds Decree). By virtue of it, all those employed beneath a given wage limit henceforth must be insured against the costs of illness by an 'Algemeen Ziekenfonds', i.e. by an officially recognised sickness fund. Dependent wives and children were included in the compulsory scheme. Those earning more than the wage limit, the self-employed and those not employed could participate on a voluntary basis. As a result, the percentage of the population insured by a sickness fund rose sharply, from 45 in 1941 to 60 in 1943. After the war, it would rise to about 70 per cent. (The additional number of people privately insured at the time is not known.) The insurance contributions were levied as a percentage of the wage, half of which was to be paid by the employee, the other half by his or her employer. Somewhat arbitrarily, the total contribution was fixed at 4 per cent.[8]

The Sickness Funds Decree had many implications. Firstly, it brought under a health insurance scheme the lowest income classes who had hitherto often been uninsured. Secondly, because of its progressive rate contributions, it imposed a rule of solidarity upon all those insured. Thirdly and not yet mentioned, it widened the coverage of the insurance beyond pre-war limits - adding hospital and dental care - and created uniformity among sickness funds in this respect. Fourthly, it imposed state supervision and control on the entire field. This was the death warrant for many disreputable commercial funds that functioned at the time. Fifthly, it brought in employers as an interested party into the arrangement. One can question the wisdom of this social innovation, but its consequences for post-war developments cannot be denied.

Of course, the Sickness Funds Decree had equally significant flaws. Most importantly, it was a workers insurance instead of a universal scheme: the self-employed and the elderly were excluded and could only take part in the voluntary insurance by paying higher, flat-rate premiums. While a circle of solidarity was drawn to include all lower-income workers (employees) and their dependants, the same circle excluded others with equally low incomes. This weakness would haunt Dutch social health insurance for a long time to come.

The Germans had several reasons for introducing a Sickness Funds Decree in The Netherlands. They clearly wished to calm the Dutch people and to lull them into believing that they had good intentions. In the back of their heads, of course, they were dreaming of a Greater German Reich, of which The Netherlands would be a province. Hence the general emphasis on 'Gleichschaltung' or equalisation. More specifically, the Germans wanted to put Dutch employers on a par with their German counterparts, i.e. tax them as heavily as employers in Germany were being taxed for the `Krankenkassen' (the German version of sickness funds). By the way:; similarities between German and Dutch social security arrangements existed long before the German Occupation, as a result of policy copying after the Bismarckian model. And there where other motives: the Sickness Funds Decree, for instance, was one more instrument in an orchestrated attempt to subject Dutch doctors and their (K)NMG to German authority. This attempt failed. The doctors refused to collaborate, stood by the side of their Jewish colleagues and more generally played an honourable role during the War. They were to gain much credit and moral authority from this afterwards.

Postwar restoration[9]

After the Liberation in May 1945, two opposing tendencies collided in the field of health insurance, as they were to do in other sectors of Dutch society. In the last years of the war, both the government in exile in London and leading figures from the resistance movement in the Netherlands had laid down their own plans for fundamental change in Dutch society, to be implemented after the Liberation. Their plans differed widely. Queen Wilhelmina, grandmother to our present Queen Beatrix and likewise in exile at the time, had even nursed slightly authoritarian fantasies of a guided democracy, led by a strong monarchy - that is by her. To her credit, she withdrew her plans in good time. More realistic plans were also drawn up in London, such as the one for the future social security system by the Van Rhijn Commission. On the other side of the North Sea, leaders of the resistance had dreamt of breaking down pre-war religious polarisation, of a unified trade union movement, and a major political realignment that would facilitate the modernisation and liberalisation of society. Where these two groups could agree was over the necessity for structural change. Soon they would meet formidable forces of restoration.

At the first post-war general election, the newly formed social democratic party, the 'Partij van den Arbeid' (PvdA, that is the Labour party) did not achieve the landslide victory that many had expected, and the Labour party achieved in Britain. Pre-war political balances of power were reproduced with surprising accuracy. Post-war governments were to be coalition governments once again; the only difference being the fact that henceforth the social democrats would be serious candidates for inclusion in cabinets. Between 1946 and 1994, Holland was governed in turn by centre-right and centre-left coalitions. (In 1994, for the first time in history a conservative-liberal-socialist coalition was forged, with some interesting though minor consequences.) Religious parties held the pivotal position throughout the period. Together with the social democrats they contributed to the rebuilding of the Dutch economy and, later, the expansion of the welfare state.

This political restoration helps to explain why in 1945 and 1946 the German Sickness Funds Decree was not revoked and replaced by another, more radical, legal arrangement. Although schemes for a national, that is, universal, insurance were being circulated and the Van Rhijn Commission had given a boost to this line of thinking, there was strong opposition from, among others, the KNMG. Not only did they reject the idea of a national insurance, a national health service and the inevitable state bullying this would bring about - imagine the horror of being a state employee! - but they also tried to revoke the Sickness Funds Decree for being too collectivist, too stifling to their profession, and too soft on their patients. General practitioners cancelled their contracts with the sickness funds. There was even an attempt by a minority of doctors to portray the upsurge in demand for medical services after the war as proof of the effeminacy that compulsory insurance schemes with proportional levies (that is, almost free) evoke in the population.[10] The moral courage many Dutch doctors had shown during the War, did not translate into an enlightened social consciousness.

Under these circumstances, the first post-war cabinet, preferring a bird in the hand to two in the bush, decided to uphold the Sickness Funds Decree. It defined the Decree as an essentially Dutch measure - which was not true - and gave it a proper legal status. The figure of Commissioner for State Supervision, at the head of the organisation, was felt to be too reminiscent of the German Occupation and was replaced by a temporary Advisory Committee, members of which were drawn from all interested parties: sickness funds; medical professions; employers; employees; and the ministry of Social Affairs. In 1949 this Committee was in turn replaced by a permanent body, the 'Ziekenfondsraad' or Sickness Fund Council, with the same fivefold representative structure. This Council was to supervise the sickness funds in The Netherlands; it was to administer the flow of monies that pertained to the funds; and it was to advise the government on social health insurance. The Sickness Fund Council would indeed play a central role in health insurance policies for half a century.

However, the very first opinion sought from Sickness Fund Council by the government concerned the future organisation of social health insurance. Ironically but not surprisingly, considering the composition of the Council, this proved to be a major stumbling block. The Council was deeply divided and in the end was not able to come up with a collective view. Annoyed by the long delays and the intractable nature of the problem, successive governments and ministers turned to the solution of other, more urgent and politically more gratifying problems.

In fact, when reading Charles Webster's The National Health Service: A Political History, we were struck by his sketch of the spirit of euphoria and consensus in Britain during and shortly after the war. 'The idea of a national health service evoked spontaneous and passionate support from all sections of the community.'[11] Aneurin skilfully tapped into this spirit, or so it seems to us, and forged his NHS in the heat of it. No such unity and enthusiasm existed in The Netherlands, at least, that is, not in the field of health care. In the field of old age provision, a similar phenomenon did occur. Willem Drees, social democrat, minister of Social Affairs (and prime minister on many occasions in the future) devised the first universal state pension scheme in The Netherlands in 1948 (the Emergency Law on Old Age Provision, later to be succeeded by the General Old Age Law). It was greeted with acclaim by all and with deep personal gratitude by the elderly. Even today Drees is revered as the greatest statesman in our modern history - probably the only one to set against Bevan as a public figure and perhaps even more universally esteemed. The 'Algemene

Ouderdomswet AOW' (i.e. the General Old Age Law) acquired the same sacrosanct status that the NHS seems to enjoy in the United Kingdom. No political party can afford to tamper with it.[12]

'Congealed power'

In an interview conducted in the course of research into the history of the Sickness Fund Council, a fellow historian, himself a member of the Council, described the Council to us as 'congealed power dating from before the war'.[13] This is a very apt characterisation. In the Sickness Fund Council, the antagonisms between the different interest groups that used to fight each other before the War were indeed 'congealed' into institutionalised consultation.

This had considerable advantages. Decisions that were somewhat less political in nature could safely be left to the Sickness Fund Council to prepare and, in practice, take. (Formally of course, important decisions always had to be made by the minister for Social Affairs.) Likewise, nasty political problems could sometimes be neutralised by putting them out to nurse with the Council. Once the long process of discussion, consultation and internal decision-making had been worked through within the Council, a high degree of commitment and co-operation by all the parties involved was guaranteed, making it much easier to guide legislation through Parliament. For politicians this corporatism held an important attraction - or temptation: it was cumbersome, slow, often undemocratic, but it guaranteed policy implementation.[14] From 1949 until the 1970s, the Sickness Fund Council fulfilled its functions quite well. Existing legislation was fine-tuned; a number of problems were solved by means of additional legislation (for example, a separate insurance scheme for the elderly); the Council took responsibility for the implementation of a major new law on Exceptional Medical Expenses in 1968 (the 'Algemene Wet Bijzondere Ziektekosten' AWBZ, a national insurance); administrative innovations were developed and implemented; a tight regime of control was exerted over the sickness funds, preventing inefficiencies. These of course were the years of economic growth - first slow, but accelerating from the 1960s onwards. It can be argued that decision-making in a corporatist, multi-party body like the Sickness Fund Council is easier under conditions of economic prosperity. Positive sum games can be played, attractive bargains can be struck, solutions can be found that satisfy all parties. Especially in the

1960s these conditions applied and within the Ziekenfondsraad the culture of consultation and corporatist decision-making flourished.

But the congealed nature of the situation also had major disadvantages. As has already been mentioned, the Sickness Fund Council proved dramatically unable to advise the government on a fully-fledged Sickness Fund Law[15] - a legislative project still to be completed after the provisional legalisation of the Sickness Funds Decree in 1945. In the end, a strong willed Roman Catholic minister of Health, Gerard Veldkamp, himself an expert in social insurance, completed the job almost single-handedly. As it happened, the Sickness Fund Law (in force from 1966) did not fundamentally diverge from the principles of the 1941 Decree. The Sickness Fund Council was maintained, albeit with numerical changes: the medical professionals lost somewhat in power, the employers' organisations and the unions gained.[16] On the whole, though, the dynamics remained the same and the label 'congealed power' was as valid as before.

The imperative of cost-containment

Another way to describe this situation could be interlocking powers who keep each other in order and thereby regulate themselves. The term stale-mate also comes to mind. In spite of its advantages it was to prove inadequate. What happened? Those familiar with health politics in other countries may already have guessed. From approximately 1973 onwards, the necessity for cost-containment forced itself onto the political agenda, and was later to transform itself into the need of retrenchment. There were two main reasons for this. First, costs of health care had been rising at least from the beginning of the nineteen-sixties.[17] And second, the great solution to all our problems: economic growth, had started to waver. The first oil crisis of 1973 was a dramatic announcement of this change of climate. The 1970s saw low levels of economic growth with rising unemployment; the beginning of the 1980s witnessed a fully-fledged economic recession and mass unemployment. The story will be all too familiar to British readers.

To make a long story short: the corporatist nature of the field of health care in The Netherlands, combined with the mixed, somewhat mosaic-like structure of Dutch health insurance, proved to be difficult to control from the point of view of cost containment. Successive governments were to find it an intractable problem. Jo Hendriks, minister of Health in a center-left coalition from 1973-1977, adopted an ambitious 'statist' strategy of restructuring, controlling, steering and regulating. This largely failed, but he did succeed in devising instruments for financial monitoring and auditing that had hitherto been lacking. His successors, especially the ministers of Health in the first two centre right cabinets led by Ruud Lubbers - a friend and admirer of Margaret Thatcher, but a far less controversial politician - put these instruments to good use, forging them into budgetary measures and constraints. They also applied a catalogue of other measures like direct prescription and referral charges. These measures met with much opposition in Parliament, among the general public and with the interested parties. Nonetheless they were pushed through. Also the government became locked in a war with the pharmaceutical interest groups which continues to this day.

This long drawn out excercise of cost containment and retrenchment soured the relationship between politicians and the field of health care. Increasingly, politicians came to resent what they perceived as non-cooperation, delaying tactics or outright obstructionism. The same phenomenon occurred in other fields. The irritations focused in particular on the labyrinth of quasi-autonomous advisory and regulatory bodies that flouished in the Netherlands. In the 1980s, a determination to remove this corporatist legacy gradually gained momentum - under the banner of 'the primacy of politics' - and in the 1990s many of the advisory and regulatory bodies were indeed abolished. The Sickness Fund Council lingered on but finally, in 1999, the fifty years of its existence came to an end. Its supervisory functions are now carried out by a 'College voor Zorgverzekeringen' (Council or Board for Care Insurances), whose members are appointed by the minister of health on the basis of their expertise. The interest groups have been thrown out, their joint 'congealed' power is finally being dissipated. At least, that is, in this particular form. It would be naive to expect them not to regroup, and in fact, they have done so. Instead of the official corporatist structures of consultation of old, new, unofficial structures have sprung up. Health insurance companies and organizations of medical professionals and hospitals have taken to meeting regularly meet behind closed doors in a so-called 'Treek-overleg', named after the splendid country estate Den Treek where the great and the good enjoy good wines and smoke fine cigars in each other's company. Jealousy apart, there is a considerable risk of market-corporatism developing to fill the gap left by the abolition of state-corporatism.[18]

The blessings of the market

And it all happened because yes, the Dutch too, were finally converted to the creed of the market. Their evangelist was not 'a maverick American systems analyst' (with thanks to Charles Webster) but he did come from Eindhoven. Wisse Dekker, chairman of the board of control of the multinational Philips Electronics (Eindhoven, NL) and therefore the obvious candidate to reorganize social health insurance in The Netherlands, presided over a Commission named after him. An important figure behind the scenes was dr. W.P.M.M. van de Ven, later to become a professor of health economics and management, who was probably the first to advocate Enthoven-like prescriptions for Dutch health insurance. In 1987 The Dekker Commission produced an influential report called Willingness to Change, advocating a combination of a universal, compulsory basic insurance with limited coverage on the one hand, with voluntary additional insurance on the other. The scheme was to be carried out by both sickness funds and private insurance companies, who were to compete against one another. In fact, the difference between the two was to melt away: Sickness funds would be permitted to compete in the market for private insurances, and private companies would be allowed to capture a share in the compulsory insurance market. (Notice that in the Dutch case the market created or enlarged is one for health care insurance companies, not one for service providers. There are provisions for managed competition between providers too, but we cannot go into them here.)

From 1991 onwards, this part of the Dekker Commission's recommendations was indeed implemented. The result was a revolution in the health insurance market and in the insurance market in general. Sickness funds quickly shook off their traditional non-profit skins and transformed themselves into 'moderne zorgverzekeraars' (modern care-insurance companies). They merged with each other and with commercial companies, and then in turn merged with general insurance companies, transforming themselves into financial conglomerates. Within eight years, the market turned into a state of proto-oligopoly. In name, there are now about thirty care insurance companies left, out of the more than one hundred that existed in 1991. In reality, the market is dominated by about eight giant conglomerates. From the point of view of willingness to change, the operation was a resounding success. From the point of view of market dynamics, the stage of free competition seems already dead and buried. The supporters of the free market are now worried about the consequences of this development. Those critical of the free market have been worried all along.

It should be pointed out, however, that the compulsory-insurance segment of the market is strongly regulated by the state. Risk selection by insurance companies is not allowed; tariffs are fixed; the services covered under the insurance are uniform, determined by the minister of health and, ultimately, by parliament. Competition and oligopolisation can only occur in the voluntary-insurance segment. It is precisely because of this that it is so difficult to assess the operation of marketisation. As the Dutch Social and Cultural Planning Bureau recently observed: 'It is a dilemma: the government pursues the goal of a controlled market for medical services, but the unwanted negative effects demand so much control that such a market cannot function.'[19]

The other part of the Dekker Commission's recommendations fared less well. The details of a universal basic insurance scheme proved to be controversial. The same minister of health who in 1991 released market forces among insurance companies, Hans Simons, could not get his plans for a basic insurance through parliament. They smelled too much of a national insurance and, to many parties and interest groups in Holland, the idea of national insurance against the costs of illness is still taboo. The new liberal-conservative-social democrat cabinets under Wim Kok (1994-present) have proclaimed a 'breathing space'. Two of the coalition partners the VVD ('Volkspartij voor Vrijheid en Democratie', liberal conservative) and the PvdA have diametrically opposed views on the issue. In the long run though, a limited basic insurance scheme for all is still the most likely outcome. Sooner or later, step by step rather than by one grand political gesture and possibly attracting very little attention, such a scheme is likely to emerge.

Some conclusions

A comparative analysis of developments in health care and health insurance in Great Britain and The Netherlands would require a book-length study.[20] Above, we merely gave a sketch of some Dutch developments and peculiarities. Immediately, both differences and similarities strike the eye. To conclude, we would like to pick up one of each.

Why is there no National Health Service in Holland? The crudest answer seems to be this:

(1) because The Netherlands had and still has an electoral system of proportional representation;
(2) because The Netherlnads had a weaker and less unified workers' or socialist movement;
(3) because the Dutch did not have the socially unifying experience of suffering and winning a just war.

Having a one-party government with a solid, left wing majority behind him and being able to build upon a community spirit that had been greatly enhanced by the War, Aneurin Bevan built the National Health Service. And of course: he was the right man on the right moment in the right place. The Dutch did have the right man: Willem Drees. But they did not have a recent unifying experience. In fact, the Dutch had undergone a profound humiliation that had divided them more than it had unified them. (We are thinking of the deportation and murder of the Jews; the brave but ineffective resistance by some; the collaboration of others; the accommodation of most.) They had a comparatively weak socialist or social democratic movement, and they had proportional representation which, in spite of its many advantages, does not lend itself easily to the implementation of grand schemes, especially not in a multi-religious and nowadays, increasingly multi-cultural, society like The Netherlands. The fact that Willem Drees did manage to legislate his Old Age Law seems to contradict what we just said. But compared to a National Health Service this was a much more modest accomplishment: there were, for one thing, no doctors needing to be bullied or bribed.

A more specific, historical factor that has also blocked initiatives towards a National Health Service in Holland was the strong position that the medical profession had obtained within the field of the sickness funds. As mentioned earlier, the Dutch Medical Society (K)NMG had very cleverly established and organized its own 'maatschappijfondsen'. By controlling them they largely controlled the field of social health insurance. Between 1949 and 1965 for example, the Sickness Fund Council was dominated by its two largest factions: the doctors and the funds. Together they held an absolute majority. But as doctors controlled the majority of the funds, they also controlled at least part of the chairs of the funds in the Sickness Fund Council, which was very clever indeed. In the long run, the power of the medical profession in Holland was broken not by their natural or class enemies, the mutual funds and the patients, but by the state. The politicians running the state needed a crisis of the welfare state in order to be convinced of its necessity. More and more, doctors nowadays work as employees of community centers, hospitals, universities, state and even commercial organizations.

Finally there is the question of the similarity, or perhaps even convergence, between the Dutch and the British situations. While reading Webster's history of the National Health Service, an institution which, we hope to have demonstrated, is fundamentally different from Dutch arrangements, we were nevertheless surprised by the many similarities. These are striking parallels in time scales in developments in Britain and Holland. Webster's three phases of 'creation and consolidation', of 'planning and reorganisation' and of 'revolution' can certainly be applied to the history of the Dutch sickness funds and perhaps to the entire Dutch health care system as well. Margaret Thatcher's supplanting of public interest quangos by advisory committees of her own ideological soul mates reminded us of the many ad hoc committees chaired by businessmen whose prescriptions we (the Dutch) have had to swallow. The Dekker Commission was only one of them, and the entire 'primacy of politics' and 'away-with-corporatism' campaign was prompted by other committees, chaired by public management gurus.

There seem to be two broad explanations for these 'processual' similarities, once again very crude ones. (1) The United Kingdom and The Netherlands have been (and are) subject to the same macro-economic and, as we now fashionably say, global constraints. We already touched upon the importance of economic growth for the functioning of corporatist consultation. Mutatis mutandis, it will be easy to point out corroding effects of the economic stagnation in the 1970s and 1980s upon different forms of consultation within the British NHS. Economic adversity tends to erode institutionalized modes of fuctioning and established configurations of power; it tends to evoke forced, statist and centralist reactions; and it tends to solicit equally forced market-oriented, decentralist strategies when these do not work. The global economy seems to drive us from prosperity to marxism, and from marxism to marketism. What comes next, we do not know. (2) There seems to be an awful lot of policy transfer going on. In different countries and in markedly different contexts, the same recipes pop up at roughly the same time. This need not surprise us. We ourselves, as academics and sociologists of medicine, are members of a global network of health care experts, of what Abram de Swaan has called an 'international expert regime' that is continually exchanging information, knowledge, insights, views, methods, terminology and also ideology. We hope that this article may contribute to their, and our, discussions.

Notes

1. The best history of the sickness funds in The Netherlands is H.C. & E.W. van der Hoeven, *Om welzijn of winst.* [For welfare or for profit.] AZIFO, (Den Haag, 1993).See also De Wit, 'Geschiedenis van de ziekenfonds- en de algemene ziektekostenverzekering' [History of the sickness funds insurance and the general health insurance.] in *De groei van de sociale verzekering in Nederland.* Vereeniging van Raden van Arbeid, (Amsterdam, 1970), pp.129-156. Many more references can be found in Bottenburg, Maarten van, Geert de Vries en Annet Mooij. *Zorg tussen staat en markt. De maatschappelijke betekenis van de Ziekenfondsraad 1949-1999.* [Care beteen state and market. The social impact of the Sickness Fund Council 1949-1999.] Walburg Pers, (Zutphen, 1999).
2. (Koninklijke) Nederlandse Maatschappij tot bevordering der Geneeskunst; the predicate `Koninklijke' [Royal] was acquired after the Second World War.
3. Together, these three categories of funds covered some 70 per cent of all those insured. We will not go into the heterogeneous lot of funds covering the other 30 per cent.
4. In the area of social sickness insurance, the protestant and the socialist (or social democratic) sections in Dutch society have tended to cooperate much more than in other areas.
5. See Cox, R.H. *The development of the Dutch welfare state. From workers' insurance to universal entitlement.* University of Pittsburg Press, (Pittsburgh/London, 1993) and Pierson, P. 'The new politics of the welfare state', *World Politics*, 48, 2 (January 1996), pp.143-179, respectively.
6. After Doorn, J.A.A. van. 'De verzorgingsmaatschappij in de praktijk.' [The welfare society in practice.] In: J.A.A. van Doorn & C.J.M. Schuyt (eds.) *De stagnerende verzorgingsstaat,* Boom, (Meppel, 1978), pp.17-47.
7. The history of the Sickness Fund Decree has been written by Hoeven, H.C. van der. *Ziekenfondsen en de Duitse bezetting. De werkelijkheid over het Ziekenfondsenbesluit 1941.* [Sickness funds and the German occupation. The truth about the Sickness Funds Decree.], Koninklijke Vermande/AZIVO, (Lelystad/Den Haag, 1989).
8. After the War, this percentage turned out to have been higher than necessary. The Dutch sickness funds collectively commanded a considerable financial reserve that helped them absorb the post-war surge in demand for medical treatment. In the nineteen-fifties, they were forced to empty the reserve by the government, whishing to keep down the insurance premiums and through them wage-costs. Bottenburg, Maarten van, Geert de Vries en Annet Mooij. *Zorg tussen staat en markt. De maatschappelijke betekenis van de Ziekenfondsraad 1949-1999.* [Care beteen state and market. The social impact of the Sickness Fund Council 1949-1999.] Walburg Pers, (Zutphen, 1999).
9. A general overview of the relationship between state and health care between 1945 and 1970 is provided by Juffermans, Paul. *Staat en gezondheidszorg in Nederland.* [State and health care in The Netherlands.] SUN, (Nijmegen, 1982).

10.   Juffermans, Paul. *Staat en gezondheidszorg in Nederland*. [State and health care in The Netherlands.] SUN, (Nijmegen, 1982), pp.184-185.

11.   Webster, Charles. *The National Health Service. A political history*, Oxford UP, (Oxford, New York, 1998), p.8.

12.   As Eelco Brinkman, the then leader of the Christian Democrats, found out in 1992. In an unwise moment of honesty during election time, he questioned tenability of the AOW. This contributed to the Christian Democrats being voted out of power for the first time in 75 years.

13.   Ele Visser, quoted in Bottenburg, Maarten van, Geert de Vries en Annet Mooij. *Zorg tussen staat en markt. De maatschappelijke betekenis van de Ziekenfondsraad 1949-1999.* [Care beteen state and market. The social impact of the Sickness Fund Council 1949-1999.] Walburg Pers, (Zutphen, 1999).

14.   This point has been stressed by Wolff, L.J. de. 'Tussen corporatisme en etatisme' [Between corporatism and etatism.], in: L.J. de Wolff (ed), *De prijs voor gezondheid. Het Centraal Orgaan Ziekenhuistarieven 1965-1982.* Ambo, (Baarn, 1984), pp.219-235.

15.   For unknown reasons, the Sickness Funds Decree became the Sickness Fund Law.

16.   Veldkamp originally whished to eliminate both the sickness funds and the medical professions from the Council, arguing that interested parties should not supervise their own functioning. He lost a political battle over this.

17.   Actually, costs had been on the rise already in the nineteen-fifties. The Sickness Fund Council had taken due notice at the time and produced reports on it with remarkable forsight. However, a strict regime of control of both wages and prices by the government kept the development within borders. Also, there was the financial reserve built up in the nineteen-forties, which could be (and was) gradually depleted.

18.   Veen, Romke van der. 'De verbouwing van Nederland', [The rebuilding of The Netherlands.] *Facta*, 6, 1 (1998), pp.14-17.

19.   SCP (Social and Cultural Planning Bureau). *Sociaal en cultureel rapport 1998.* [Social and cultural report 1998.] SCP, (Rijswijk, 1998), p.338.

20.   Compare Glaser, William. Health politics: lessons from abroad. In: Theodor J. Litman & Leonard S. Robins (eds.) *Health politics and policy.* John Wiley & Sons, (New York, 1984), pp.305-338, and Flynn, Rob. 'Restructuring health systems: a comparative analysis of England and The Netherlands' in: Michael Hill (ed.), *New agenda in the study of the policy process.* Harvester Wheatsheaf, (New York, 1993), pp.57-87

12. The Politics of Health in Scotland after Devolution

CHRIS NOTTINGHAM

Anyone who found it impossible to sleep without reading something on Scottish identity would have no reason to feel anxiety for the next decade or so. An exaggerated and, it must be said, authentically British, tendency to self-absorption has produced a literature that is comprehensive to the point of self-parody. However, while the matter of 'Scottishness' has been worried near to death, the implications for public policy of the further institutionalisation of that identity have escaped relatively lightly. It was not to be expected that the main parties in the referendum campaign would go into detail of how the new dimension would affect policy. The parties offered little more than the conventional shopping lists. Opponents of devolution found it more, but in the event, not very, productive to warn of the constitutional consequences of concessions to nationalist sentiment. For Nationalists the connection between a 'natural' political community and good public policy is an article of faith, beyond any need for detailed investigation: all that was wrong about devolution was that it did not go far enough. It fell to the parties most closely associated with the campaign for devolution to make the positive case. They did indicate a range of generalised potential gains but their arguments rested essentially on the general proposition that a focus of democratic accountability in Edinburgh was simply bound to increase the likelihood of an effective and popular public policy. Labour's Scottish Secretary effectively avoided the barbed question of precisely what he would be able to accomplish as First Minister after July 1 1999 that was not possible before.[1]

Eight months in the situation is not much clearer. Scottish Conservatives have apparently accepted the logic of the continuing run of electoral defeats and begun to distance themselves from both their past and some of the British party's current policies.[2] Nationalists have mounted a few skirmishes but have not as yet made much impression. There is division in their ranks as to how temporary a halt on the road to formal independence devolution should be, but they can afford to wait. The

173

position of main opposition party in a new institution is a relatively comfortable one and theirs is essentially a case waiting for an issue. But for the friends of the devolution settlement the problems are pressing. The two parties most closely associated with constitutional change, now harnessed together in government, are still in urgent need of a public policy which will begin to stabilise the settlement. To achieve this the policy must fulfil three requirements. It must be distinctively Scottish, in that it demonstrates the benefits of devolution itself; it must be capable of developing along lines that do not immediately solidify into zero sum confrontation with London over powers or financial resources, and thus empower the nationalist opposition; and it must be seen to be at least no less effective than what has gone before. While the Scottish electorate supports the new arrangements it is clear that their support is not unconditional.

Health is likely be one of the key areas where this challenge will have to be met. The performance of the executive in health matters will almost certainly have a major bearing on the development of the devolution policy as a whole. The fact that Labour is the lead partner in the coalition, and health is Labour's issue by tradition and choice suggests this, but the prominence of health is also a matter of the constitutional arrangements themselves. Health is one of the main matters reserved to the Scottish Parliament and Executive and one where public interest is consistent and, on occasion, intense. Another obvious way of expressing the importance of health for post-devolutionary politics is in terms of the share of public expenditure it commands. Health accounts for 32 per cent of the Scottish Office's expenditure with current changes likely to push the proportion even higher.[3] On such a basis health will never be far from the Executive's concerns and the Parliament's Health Committee is likely to be a popular choice for ambitious MSPs. Similarly the significance of health in employment terms should not be forgotten. In times when investments producing a few hundred jobs are treated as political triumphs the significance of nearly 140,000 people directly employed within the NHS in Scotland needs little emphasis. The centrality of health in Scottish politics can also be expressed in terms of striking, and much discussed, morbidity and mortality figures.[4] Scottish distinctiveness may be problematical in some areas but here it is clear and unequivocal. Life expectancy for both men and women is two years lower than in England and Wales. Even when the comparison is made with the English regions, which are poorer than Scotland, a gap remains. Scotland leads Western Europe in rates of premature death from heart disease, cancer, strokes and even suicide.

Glasgow has an adult mortality rate, which is 30 per cent above the UK average.[5] It is scarcely surprising that such statistics have attracted the attention of political reformers as well as public health campaigners. The Scottish Constitutional Convention (SCC) argued that 'the Scots are not an inherently unhealthy people'. While there is no definitive understanding of the underlying causes of Scotland's poor health record it has become an article of faith with reformers that a Scottish Parliament represents the best way forward. In their document of 1995 the SCC suggested a direct relationship between constitutional reform and good health policy. Parliament, it argued, will be able to arrange the organisation, funding and policy of health provision to deliver the sort of health service Scotland wants. It will be able to decide the best ways of supporting family life; of providing care for people with handicaps, illnesses or disabilities, the elderly and for children in need; and it will be able to ensure that local authorities and health authorities co-operate to maintain and improve these services.[6]

The apparent intractability of Scotland's problems, it suggested, would disappear with the application of 'the principles of democratic accountability and decentralisation.' Constitutional change would release a new creativity: 'In particular a broader vision of public health would allow a far more effective attack on the many factors contributing to preventable ill health.' It is easy enough to pick holes in this case: did it, for instance do justice to the many organisations and individuals in Scotland who have battled with such problems for years to suggest that they had failed and that a single change was all that was needed to produce success? Did it not tend to overburden a new political institution with a massive weight of unrealistic expectation? However it is impossible to deny that Scotland's health record has taken on a totemic political status. This was reinforced by the debate about the delivery of health care, which played a large part in the development of opinion in that twenty year inter-referenda period, during which constitutional change became an inevitability. In Scotland it became almost automatic to dismiss post 1979 political changes as alien impositions; health care reforms in particular were seen as having no roots in Scottish experience or need. The SCC captured the popular wisdom in arguing the *Working for Patients* reforms were 'prompted mainly by service pressures in England and in particular London', and as such their failure in Scotland was inevitable: 'Many of the problems these reforms set out to address remain unsolved … morale has suffered.'[7] Conservative policies on health did much to alienate the party from the mainstream of

Scottish sentiment and precipitate them down the slide to the point where they lost their last Westminster representatives in 1997. It has become commonplace on the left and centre of Scottish public debate, to present devolution as a final chance to save the NHS, the most cherished British institution. Changes in Scottish health policy have thus been widely attributed to English influence, 'Thatcherism', and the neglect of an Anglo centric Parliament. By implication, the way forward should now be clear.

Devolution: the weight of expectation.

Given the devastating blows, which all sections of the left and centre of British politics sustained in the years after 1979, an immense weight of expectation was bound to attach itself to anything which threatened the Conservative hegemony. The feelings of frustration were all the greater in Scotland as changes were introduced without visible support. So, although the effects of change, particularly in health, were more limited than elsewhere in the United Kingdom; partly because of the operations of the Scottish Office which even in Conservative hands served as a defender of the Scottish status quo; the sense that they were an alien imposition was intense among professionals and public alike. The demand for devolution, the demand that it should no longer be possible for central government to operate in defiance of Scottish opinion, came to focus the hopes of all manner of reformers. Yet while Scottish activists of the left and centre were frustrated, the ubiquity of anti-Conservative sentiment protected then from the despair which drove the New Labour project in England. Although excluded from power, they never experienced that withering of support among traditional supporters which provided the impetus for figures such as Philip Gould.[8] It was possible to believe that if a means could be found of enabling the majority will to assert itself there was still life in traditional redistributive politics. At the same time, and for similar reasons, there developed a state of mind, which did not consider too closely the possibility that unpalatable changes might have more complex causes. Many were happy to see such alterations as the rise of managerialism in the health service as originating in political will and as such, removable by a contrary will.

Inevitably a series of very different projections of the post-devolution political community took shape. Sometimes the 'settled will of the Scottish people' pointed to a future in which the traditional virtues of community would be restored. Scotland's communitarian culture would form the basis for the restoration of a politics of redistribution. Scotland still stood where she did. To others, however, this settled will would encompass a benign modernity. Where Westminster was characterised by negativity, adversarialism, obfuscation, and elitism, Edinburgh would be outward looking, inclusive, woman-friendly, constructive and polite.

A devolved health policy came to bear a burden expectation that was intense but not always precise or internally consistent. For the SCC devolved health politics would be one of the pillars of the new consciousness: 'It is easy to envisage health questions and health debates in the Parliament becoming compelling listening to professionals and public alike.'[9] Similarly it envisaged the reversal of past neglects: 'a broader vision of public health would allow a far more effective attack on the many factors contributing to preventable ill health.' This latter theme has been taken up enthusiastically. Alysson Pollock has argued that the most critical issue facing the devolved parliament is whether it will devote its energies to the redistributive measures, which she sees as the critical element in the fight against health inequalities.[10] Steven Maxwell, Assistant Director of the Scottish Council for Voluntary Organisations, has taken strong issue with those who are pessimistic about the prospects: 'If even half the hopes of the most zealous reformers are fulfilled the Scottish Parliament will operate more as a catalyst to a civic process of change, then as a traditional monopolistic legislature.'[11] Yet there is a striking contrast between the scale of Maxwell's general hopes and that of his specific proposals. He suggests, for example that the Parliament should use its limited tax raising powers to give Scottish pensioners a one hundred pounds Christmas bonus or to top up child benefit payments. Such ideas may be attractive in themselves but there must be a practical doubt as to whether they would justify the considerable expenditure of political energy involved or whether other courses of action might not more effectively produce the desired results.

It is easy to see why those campaigning against health inequalities should seize on the devolved systems in Scotland and Wales, as both seem to be the remaining repositories of majority support for traditional social policies. It is not, however, at all clear whether or how these opinions can be transformed into practical policy. The basic case of those concerned to rectify health inequalities has, after all, less to do with the health care measures, which are within the Parliament's remit, than social security, taxation and public expenditure ones, which are not. There is the option of raising more money in Scotland and devoting it to supplementary policies in such areas. However the fact that the tax varying powers of the Scottish Parliament are exclusively attached to income might prove unfortunate in this respect. If the executive were to raise the 3 per cent additional tax, which is possible, and devote it to removing health inequalities they would run the risk of attacks on all fronts. Nationalists would certainly claim that Scotland was being asked to pay for the consequences of London's long neglect. Conservatives would point to possible harmful effects on inward investment. Both would find an audience among Scottish income tax payers. Moreover the amount raised; at around £700 million would not be of the order to produce any immediate visible effect on what everyone agrees is a deeply rooted problem. The alternative is for the Parliament and Executive to argue for additional public funds from the UK budget. This however looks as though it will become increasingly difficult, for English MPs, particularly those from the poorer regions are inevitably watching the situation closely. Scotland currently spends around 23 per cent more on health per head of population that the UK average.[12] That is where agreement ceases. Some argue that the additional funding reflects 'the greater burden of ill health in Scotland and the need to deliver services to sparsely populated areas.'[13] Allyson Pollock suggests that if the population based formula on which the distribution of public expenditure is currently allocated (the famous Barnett Formula) were replaced by one based on need Scotland might even possibly qualify for more.[14] Jennifer Dixon disagrees. In her sensitively titled article 'Is the English NHS underfunded?', she argues that it is historical factors, that is decades of political horse trading, rather than special needs that are responsible for this imbalance, and moreover Scotland seems to achieve very little with its additional funds.[15] Others make the same point in a less conciliatory spirit. Sarah Hogg, formerly policy adviser to John Major, produced 'England gets tired of constant gifts to Scotland'.[16] The passions and interests involved in the debate suggest that any settlement will be politically rather than intellectually determined. If devolution has achieved nothing else it has certainly increased English sensitivities towards Scottish public expenditure. Even with the best will in the world one cannot imagine MP's from the poorer English regions failing to make the case for their own constituents in any future debate about additional Scottish funding, however benign the purpose.

Mobilising Support

The most optimistic supporters of devolution rest their hopes on a particular interpretation of the character of the Scottish electorate. If there were a body of settled support for a redistributive policy, as they assume, it would certainly make it easier for the Executive to face the other difficulties. There is some evidence to support such an interpretation. Scottish voters have certainly shown consistent and, in UK terms, disproportionate, support for parties broadly resistant to Conservative hostility to public expenditure. Hazell and Jervis go further:

> The traditional culture in Scotland and Wales is strongly 'communitarian'. Devolution is seen as a chance to reassert and build on this culture, and the health service will provide a highly visible test of the ability to do this.[17]

The British Election Survey of 1997 did find clear, if not always deep, differences between Scottish and English voters.[18] Brown, McCrone and Paterson note that differences tend to be greatest in those areas, such as general attitudes to taxation and redistribution, which do not fall within the remit of the devolved Parliament.[19] Their conclusion is that 'Scottish policy preferences are not very distinct from those in the rest of Britain. Insofar as there are differences, however, they do put Scotland more to the left politically than elsewhere.' However they suggest that the differences that do exist probably arise from, 'links between certain policy positions and Scottish national identity.'[20] This suggests that it might be better to see Scottish popular collectivism as a historically developed tactic related to securing maximum advantage within UK politics and that it might be more difficult to mobilise it in support of redistributive policies of a devolved executive within a Scottish framework.

The most comfortable and least divisive definitions of Scottishness are always ones which revolve around non-Englishness, and Edinburgh politicians will always face the temptation of presenting themselves as embattled defenders of the national interest. This is a familiar and comfortable line and has been a major route to success in Scottish politics for many decades. The office of Secretary of State for Scotland has always demanded something above the party political.[21] If devolution though is to mean little more than a continuation of an old policy by other means it raises the question as to why have devolution in the first place. If the game is one of sorting out Scottish internal differences and then presenting a united front in UK bargaining the thing might even be better done out of the limelight. The new openness is only a virtue if it is directed, as the constitutional idealists hope, to making qualitative changes in the Scottish political community. If the old ways are coupled to greater transparency, it is possible to foresee difficulties in establishing a unified Scottish position as well as in advancing that position at UK level. The worst outcome, at least from the point of view of those who wish to see the current settlement work, would be institutionalised division in Edinburgh around the question of who was most adept at promoting the Scottish interest, thus provoking automatic resistance in London.

The complexities of health policy

Health policy, then, will be one of the main areas in which the devolved institutions will have to demonstrate their usefulness. A credible showing here will be necessary for the plausibility of the whole policy. However health is one of the more complex and politically sensitive areas and the difficulties involved in producing acceptable and efficient policies are great. At the deepest level, health questions in modern industrial states have a particular bearing on questions of statehood and citizenship. In recent years, as the states of the developed world have sought to limit their responsibilities, by abolition or more usually redistribution, health has nearly always proved to be the area of greatest resistance. Health and welfare questions are perhaps the only ones that can still be relied upon to create genuine debate about the relative responsibilities of the state, the professional, the family and the individual. Entitlements to benefit, particularly health benefit, are at the heart of modern citizenship. Whereas in the nineteenth century the debate about citizenship revolved around the entitlement to vote, in the second half of the twentieth century such debates were largely conducted in terms of rights to benefits. Both the moral and operational boundaries of political communities are deeply influenced by entitlements to benefit. Similarly they can be seen as the lynch pin of the legitimacy of the modern state. Health policy will thus be unable to escape a prominent, and potentially explosive, role in the development of the whole devolution settlement. Moreover any changes which the executive feels to be desirable will have to be implemented without compromising service delivery. In their demands for safety and certainty, and their acute sensitivity to failure, Scottish patients are no different from their English counterparts.

Neither is health an area in which it is particularly easy for states to impose their own priorities. While states have heavy and unavoidable responsibilities in the area there are factors which heavily restrict their field of choice. Health policy makers in all modern states face the financial and service challenges posed by ageing populations, ever more expensive technologies, rising citizen expectations increasingly reinforced by the ease of international comparison, and plunging levels of deference on the part of the public towards health care professionals. Running a health care state in a modern industrial society involves maintaining a semblance of balance between commercial and professional interests operating at both national and international levels. Moreover this must be accomplished in the context of public expenditure stringency and in the realisation that failure here is liable to be punished far more heavily than elsewhere.[22]

There are also reasons to suppose that the NHS, which dealt fairly effectively with the problems of political economy encountered in its earlier years, is less successfully geared to coping with the current situation. One of the key difficulties for working politicians is its tendency to keep service and financial issues in the forefront of political debate on an almost day to day basis. Tony Blair's recent pledge, or aspiration, to increase levels of health care spending in the UK up to the European average, fits into a familiar pattern in which public reaction to service failure in the NHS demands prime ministerial intervention and the promise of additional funding. Developing a devolved element, or indeed any reform, becomes additionally difficulty in an area where even the maintenance of stability and public calm requires constant vigilance and political effort.

There is also a certain confusion over the NHS within British political culture, which adds to the difficulties. Most people claim to support it but it is not clear exactly what it is that they are supporting. Most accounts suggest that it is the principle that is popular but even this is ambiguous. For some it might be the collective principle, the benefits, practical and moral, that come to everyone from the fact that there is nobody in the society who is denied necessary health care. For others the principle which the NHS embodies might be a more self interested one: the NHS guarantees treatment without the bother and pain of paying for it individually. This interpretation of principle may be somewhat elusive, in that individuals would be more reluctant to talk about it, but this does not mean it should be discounted, particularly in a society where the cash nexus is becoming ever more central in the provisions of other goods and services.

There are also ambiguities connected with the scope of the NHS. The blanket promise to respond to 'need' will always leave room for interpretation. Conservative government promises that the NHS was 'safe' with them did not prevent the curtailment of optician services or long term care for the elderly any more than Labour promises of a more vigorous defence of the NHS seems to involve their reinstatement.

However, the ambiguity which surrounds the NHS does not always serve to make life easier for politicians. Indeed it may make it an even more potent source of danger. While it may prove relatively easy to build on some elements of the current institutional separation between the NHS in Scotland and England, any effective political separation could prove much more elusive. At the moment patients denied a particular treatment in Glasgow will feel a sense of grievance, and be able to mobilise that grievance, if they learn that it is available in Bristol or Cardiff. In this sense a UK wide NHS remains a political fact of life. This has strong implications for future change. For example the Government is currently looking to the National Institute for Clinical Excellence for authoritative decisions on which treatments and drugs are effective (or is it cost effective?) and hence should be available under the NHS. By this means it hopes to contain the political damage that comes from explicit rationing and, in particular the regional anomalies which currently cause difficulties. Yet NICE decisions will only apply in England and Wales. Scotland has its own institution for performing the same task, the Scottish Health Technology Assessment Centre.[23] This situation might serve as a measure of how far devolution could progress. Could we forsee NICE recommending the prescribing of a drug to English and Welsh patients, while SHTAC was denying it to Scots? The ultimate decision rests with the respective ministers, but it is difficult to see circumstances in which they could accept such differences.

The political complexities of the NHS do not stop there. Its most principled supporters assume a status for the Service beyond the limitations imposed by economic circumstances or other policy objectives. This has led campaigners for devolution, along with many on the left and centre of British politics, to claim that the NHS was more secure and satisfactory before the Thatcher government's reforms. This may be useful rhetorically but it provides little guidance for future action. At one level it may simply be a matter of some choices no longer being available, except at costs, which are currently politically unacceptable for anyone. At another it clearly involves a defective version of the 'golden age'. While principles might have been secure, levels of service would no longer be tolerable. If one could miraculously transfer a modern day patient into a ward in the heyday of the NHS they would probably be suing in the European Court of Human Rights by the time the night shift came on duty. Any appreciation of the NHS is unrealistic which does not take account of constant change, some of it at least, designed to accommodate the developing demands and sensitivities of patients. Professionals too would have their difficulties. It is well to remember, as we have sought to do in this volume, that, along with the benign principle, the early decades of the NHS could be characterised by student nurses on a derisory wage, exposed to the most cramped training regime, and subject to intrusive disciplinary rules; or equally by underpaid qualified nurses whose talents were routinely undervalued and underused. We could also mention low paid ancillary workers, marked variations in quality of treatment masked by the absence of effective scrutiny of professionals and institutions, patients expected to accept whatever was deemed appropriate without question, or even geriatric wards and long stay mental institutions where treatment was free but conditions often dismal. If it did seem less problematical to deliver an acceptable standard of health care this was partly because in the 'golden years' there were far fewer things that any service could perform. Discussions of health politics which fail to take account of developing medical technology and rising expectation can never be realistic.

Devolution then, can be treated in isolation neither in practice nor theory. It must be seen as one process of change in the midst of many. Scottish voters and patients may welcome aspects of a devolved NHS but they will not forgo other benefits. A Scottish Executive will have to deliver a health service, which is improving at the same rate as the equivalent services in other parts of the UK, even as it is becoming more Scottish. This is a source of difficulty, but it might also be an opportunity.

What then, is possible?

While it is possible to suggest that reformers have tended been too optimistic we should not conclude that no beneficial change will be possible. The margins may be tighter, the possibilities fewer and more restricted, and the macro political problems more intractable, but there may still be scope for the new institutions to demonstrate their usefulness. One thing which the current Executive must resist is the temptation to become the keepers of the holy grail of old Labour. They must recognise the current effective limits of political choice both in London and in Edinburgh.

Perhaps instead of demanding a redistributive fiscal regime they should work on health inequalities by initially embracing such things as Health Action Zones. They are not as has been pointed out a real substitute for a national policy but success in such ventures could open the possibility for further developments: the New Labour mantra of 'what matters is what works' does have its permissive side.

The prime asset which the Scottish Executive has at its disposal is the greater coherence of Scotland as a health policy community and its opportunity to use that asset is provided by the context of continual change within which all health care states currently find themselves. Here the suggestions of the SCC could prove to be much more realistic. It argued:

> Parliament ... will be able to decide the best ways of supporting family life, of providing care with people with handicaps illnesses or disabilities, the elderly and for children in need; and it will be able to ensure that local authorities and health authorities co-operate to maintain and improve these services.[24]

This suggests a strategy of identifying weaknesses and offering solutions from within the powers currently available. A widely recognised deficiency in the operations of the NHS has been its tendency to encourage organisational apartheid. The more progressive local authorities such as Glasgow which had assumed comprehensive responsibilities in the field of health, as Marguerite Dupree points out in this volume, were clearly the losers in the settlement of 1948 and ever since co-operation between social and health services has been restricted. The Executive could ride the rhetoric of Scottish collectivism, create a sense of impatience, and highlight, exploit and institutionalise the shorter lines of communication, existing intimacies and networking possibilities available in a devolved system. This is a particularly opportune moment, for some of the barriers which have hindered co-operation in the past are weaker. The medical profession which, as David Player illustrates above, was once opposed to local authority involvement in health matters is no longer so. Similarly, if there ever were grounds of characterising doctors as custodians of an intractable 'medical model' of health they are surely weaker now than at any time since the creation of the NHS. Medical school syllabuses and the British Medical Journal provide ample evidence of that. Similarly the old ideal of the medical man as independent professional with a monopoly on decisions about medical care is in recession. Such disparate factors as the gradual erosion of demarcation lines between doctors and nurses, NHS Direct, the managerial erosion of clinical autonomy, the steady reduction of freedom in prescribing, assertive patients, and ever more stringent clinical audit have all played their part. The decline of clinical autonomy in the health service and of formal political accountability in local government in favour of the growth of managerialism in both, has increased the possibility of multi-agency co-operative action between the two sectors. Anyone who thinks this is little more than Blairite rhetoric would do well to look at the paper which Chris Spry, the Chief Executive of the Greater Glasgow Health Board, delivered to the conference on post-devolution health services.[25] This is in part a matter of an intelligent administrator demonstrating that he knows which way the wind blows, but is much more a reflection of the impatience which many professional mangers and administrators have felt on coming up against organisational divisions and professional domination. There is a wave here which the Executive could ride.

There are then, possibilities. They arise from identifying rectifiable weakness in the current performance of the NHS and seizing opportunities which arise from the continuous process of change to which all health care regimes are currently subject. The aim should be to work within existing constraints to maintain the rate of improvement in health care services while securing visible, though incremental improvements in other areas. Given the emotional attachment of many in Scotland towards the remote areas it should be possible to use the post devolutionary situation to create imaginative policies, possibly along the lines advocated by John Curnow in this volume. Health Action Zones will never satisfy those who believe in large-scale redistribution but it may prove possible to use these and similar initiatives, in the context of new organisational co-operation, to demonstrate the possibilities of improvement.

Conclusion

In general the debate over health reform in post-devolution Scotland has been too much dominated by a strain of reforming 'whiggism'. There has been too much inclination to present devolution as an experiment based on clear research questions and susceptible to clear conclusions. The question should not be 'will devolution work?' but rather 'what will be the effect on the system of the introduction of a devolved Parliament and Executive?'. 'New dawns' are rhetorical not historical. Much of what happens will inevitably reflect what went on before. MSPs may in some respects operate in a different way from their Westminster brothers and sisters but not in all ways. They will be open when things are going well and far less so when they are not. They will find it easier to accept participation from outside groups when it seems to aid them, but they will seek to resist it when it becomes uncomfortable. The sheer size of the NHS in Scotland, the fact that it is so integral to the daily life of the society, and the fact that it is interwoven in complex patterns of public expectation, suggest that heroic changes are neither desirable nor possible. In any case an over-ambitious policy would quickly settle into a zero sum stalemate with London, which would be of no service to the friends of the devolution settlement.

Yet if the goals are realistic, if the energies of health care professionals can be harnessed in new ways and their good will restored and if changes are made strategically within the policy frameworks which match international forces and the guidelines of central government, then there is the probability of demonstrable improvement. The destiny of any plans made by the devolved institutions will not, of course, lie solely in their own hands. Much will evidently depend on the success of the UK Government in both the health and other sectors. Health care systems are subject to common influences and beset by common problems and co-operation will become even more essential both within and outside the UK. In any case it would be a great pity if international factors were seen as entirely negative. While the requirements to remain competitive in the global economy do require Governments to be visibly prudent it is equally the case that the pressure to attract inward investment does require an effective public health system and a modern and accessible system of health care. We should never fall into the habit of thinking effective health policies are simply rewards for economic efficiency.

However, if Scotland is able to share in an improving, better funded health service at national level the opportunities to exploit specifically Scottish strengths in imaginative ways will be all the greater. Perhaps this might involve some radical experimentation with the deployment of health service personnel, possibly by basing some NHS clinics around the place of work rather than the place of residence. Much might develop on the basis of greater co-operation between social and health services. Perhaps Scotland might take the lead in encouraging nurses and doctors to take on greater managerial roles thus demonstrating the point that the effective use of resources is integral to the process of caring. The reception of the Arbuthnott report suggests that an imaginative debate could develop on the deployment of resources within the NHS in Scotland. The fact tht the representative of Greater Glasgow questioned Arbuthnot's decision to transfer resources to areas whose special needs were measured by remoteness rather than deprivation is not a sign of failure but could herald a growing maturity of the devolved institutions.[26] The test of a parliament is not that it inhibits debate but that it produces a final decision which has a degree of authority.

It must also be borne in mind that not all avenues of change will prove productive. Differences between Labour's organisational white papers for England and Scotland seemed greater when they were first published than they do today. It now seems more likely that primary care co-operatives, largely because of a coincidence of professional pressures and the need to maintain cost effectiveness, will evolve in a direction not too dissimilar from Primary Care Groups in England.[27] Common pressures do tend to propel individuals in the same direction. Nothing is to be gained by assuming Scottish differences are greater than they are. The extreme faith in traditional democratic forms which some members of the SCC displayed is a case in point. Scots voted in numbers for devolution but this does not mean that they have any great faith in politicians. The early struggles of the Parliament to establish itself in the face of adverse public reaction to salaries, holidays and the cost of the new parliament building should cure anyone of that delusion. A Scottish electorate is no more likely to be satisfied with purely political controls of government agencies than any other.

Nothing is to be gained by pretending that all that has happened in UK health politics sine 1979 was the personal property of Mrs. Thatcher or that it was all dysfunctional. The systems of direct regulation and clinical governance, of management techniques such as league tables and audit do provide a means of making the health services more responsive than they previously were. They have their flaws but it is difficult to foresee their abolition. Labour's major historical defeat over nationalised industries must be seen for what it was; a huge popular rejection of formal political control. Few people would feel that the current regulatory arrangements for the former public utilities were ideal, but fewer could be found to argue that they did not represent some advance on the previous system of ministerial control. It may be the case that under the *Working for Patients* reforms that acute trusts were, in the SCC's words, 'driven into wasteful competition', but it must also be recognised that such initiatives did seek to address acknowledged problems; to undermine complacency and insinuate notions of value for money into a service often characterised by inefficiencies and inertia. Anyway Sam Galbraith the previous Scottish health minister and his successor Susan Deacon have made it explicit that return to a professionally driven service with political oversight is one option which the Scottish Parliament will not be invited to consider. However the decline in public esteem that has been suffered by politicians, and the (far more minor) one suffered by doctors might convince both that co-operation might be in both their interests. The demand for a greater interaction between the Parliament and the representatives of outside organisations which the SCC presented in idealist terms, might in the light of the above be regarded as the most practical of political proposals. The Parliament would be wise to incorporate representatives of the NHS. This would decrease its freedom of action in some respects but greatly increase it power to shape events overall.

Post devolution politics will not be easy. The wider political battle will often overwhelm careful policy initiatives and there are many potential pitfalls. The whole question of financing the NHS in Scotland is becoming one where only party political 'truths' have relevance. Similarly it is undoubtedly the case that the actual constitutional arrangements are fragile and a potential source of all manner of legal and political conflicts. There is the established 'West Lothian Question' and the brand new assertion by the Court of Session, in response to an injunction over Lord Watson's bill against hunting with dogs, that the decisions of the new Parliament are subject to judicial review in a way which the decisions of Westminster are not. It must also be remembered that politics is largely a tribal game. Even if the devolved Executive does come up with an imaginative policy options in health it will convince few of it opponents. Separatists will see success, as they would see failure, as a reason to plough on to independence. Old Labour forces will see success as evidence that the timidity of the Executive was misplaced and of the ripeness of the time for a full frontal assault on New Labour in London.

The devolved Executive has a difficult path to walk. They must develop new lines but not at the expense of discarding all the old ones. They must still make a clear show of defending Scotland's interests within the UK, which is likely to prove more rather than less difficult in the coming years, while at the same time demonstrating that Scotland's interests are best defended on the basis of a degree of autonomy within the Union. Health issues are important and may, as argued here offer a possibility of constructive policy options that might help square political circles. However such initiatives will always run the risk of being overwhelmed by some unforeseen tidal wave of political sentiment. Wales is already on its second post devolution leader because of, or at least on the pretext of, the way the

Treasury distributes EU grants. The first shots in a similar campaign in Scotland have already been fired. From what we know of post-devolution politics so far anything seems possible and no one can really say whether, or indeed how, the new institutions will establish themselves. Who would have predicted the strange cocktail of issues which have already fluttered into life? Some have been predictable such as the turf war between the First Minister and the Secretary of State for Scotland, or the several allegations of 'sleaze'. Some such as the troubles over Section 28 have been surprising. Perhaps one lesson from the last was that it does not do to assume too much about opinion in post-devolution Scotland. Clearly we shall hear a good deal more about the Barnett formula. The friends of devolution and the coalition partners alike will hope that it proves possible to squeeze in some constructive policy initiatives, but who can tell? A week in devolved politics is an even longer time.

Notes

1. See Peter Jones, 'A Start to a New Song: the 1997 Devolution Referendum Campaign.' *Scottish Affairs*, no. 21, Autumn 1997 and Charles Pattie et als., 'The 1997 Scottish Referendum: An Analysis of the Results' *Scottish Affairs*, no.22, Winter 1998.

2. See for example, 'Scots Tories reject English view on financing of NHS' *The Herald*, 2 April 1999.

3. Scottish Office Department of Health, *Scottish Health Statistics, 1996*, (Edinburgh,1997).

4. Drever F. and Whitehead M., *Health Inequalities*, London: Office for National statistics, 1997.

5. Scottish Office Department of Health, *Working Together for a Healthier Scotland*, Cm 3854, (Edinburgh, February 1998).

6. Scottish Constitutional Convention document of 1995 quoted in Colin Currie, *Health and a Scottish Parliament. A Report of a participatory conference*, (Edinburgh,1997) p.6.

7. Currie, *Health and a Scottish Parliament*, p.8.

8. See Philip Gould, *The Unfinished Revolution*, (London, 1998), particularly pp.19-37.

9. Currie, *Health and a Scottish Parliament*, p.10.

10. Allyson Pollock, 'Devolution and Health: challenges for Scotland and Wales', *BMJ* vol 318 1 May 1999, pp.1195-1198.

11. Stephen Maxwell, 'Social Policy and the Scottish Parliament: A Response to Richard Parry", *Scottish Affairs*, no.21, Autumn 1997, and for a less optimistic view, Richard Parry, 'The Scottish Parliament and Social Policy', *Scottish Affairs*, no.20, Summer 1997.

12.   Sam Galbraith, quoted in 'Health to get a higher priority in post-devolution Scotland' BMJ 1999; 318, p.80.

13.   Sam Galbraith, quoted in 'Health to get a higher priority in post-devolution Scotland' BMJ 1999; 318, p. 80.

14.   Allyson Pollock, 'Devolution and Health: challenges for Scotland and Wales', *BMJ* vol 318 1999, pp.1195-1198.

15.   Jennifer Dixon, Sarah Inglis, Rudolf Klein, 'Is the English NHS underfunded?' *BMJ* 1999; 318, pp.522-526.

16.   Sarah Hogg, 'England gets tired of constant gifts to Scotland', *The Independent*, 20 December 1998.

17.   Robert Hazell and Paul Jervis, *Devolution and Health*, Nuffield Trust, (London,1998) , p.12.

18.   British Election Survey of 1997. Data Archive Essex University.49 per cent of English respondents were in favour of selection for secondary education as opposed to 27 per cent of Scots. 31 per cent of English respondents thought government should encourage the growth of private medicine as opposed to 27 per cent of Scots.

19.   Alice Brown, David McCrone and Lindsay Paterson, Politics and Society in Scotland,Macmillan 1998.

20.   Alice Brown, David McCrone and Lindsay Paterson, Politics and Society in Scotland,Macmillan 1998, p.117.

21.   Richard Parry, 'Towards a Democratised Scottish Office?' *Scottish Affairs*, September 1993, and for a historical perspectice, Ian Levitt, *The Scottish Office : depression and reconstruction, 1919-1959*, Scottish History Society, 1992.

22.   For a recent account see Michael Moran, Governing the health care state. A comparative study of the United Kingdom, the United States and Germany. (Manchester, 1999).

23.   See 'Scotland's way to guarantee quality' *BMJ* 2000; 320, p.78 and for an insight into the potential for confusion see Arthur Morris, 'BMJ should stop confusing its readers over national differences', *BMJ* 1999:318, p.1221.

24.   Currie, *Health and a Scottish Parliament,* p.6.

25.   Chris Spry, 'NHS Boards under the New Parliament'. Paper delivered to the *Scottish Parliament and the NHS* Conference, 8 December 1998.

26.   Chris Spry argued before the Scottish Parliament Health Committee that the Arbuthnott proposals would mean a '22 per cent reduction in services like physiotherapy, district nursing and health visiting' in Glasgow. Alan MacDermid, 'Health chief tells of budget concerns', *The Herald*, 28 October 1999.

27.   For a discussion which emphasises the uncertainties in the situation see, Jane Hopton and David Heaney, 'Towards primary care groups. The development of local health care cooperatives in Scotland.' *BMJ* 1999, 318, pp.1185-1187.

Index